Public Health in America

This is a volume in the Arno Press series

PUBLIC HEALTH IN AMERICA

Advisory Editor

Barbara Gutmann Rosenkrantz

Editorial Board

**Leona Baumgartner
James H. Cassedy
Arthur Jack Viseltear**

See last pages of this volume
for a complete list of titles.

The New Public Health

HIBBERT WINSLOW HILL

ARNO PRESS

A New York Times Company

New York / 1977

Editorial Supervision: JOSEPH CELLINI

———•⦿•———

Reprint Edition 1977 by Arno Press Inc.

Reprinted from a copy in
   The University of Illinois Library

PUBLIC HEALTH IN AMERICA
ISBN for complete set: 0-405-09804-9
See last pages of this volume for titles.

Manufactured in the United States of America

———•⦿•———

Library of Congress Cataloging in Publication Data

Hill, Hibbert Winslow, 1871-1947.
   The new public health.

   (Public health in America)
   Reprint of the ed. published by Macmillan, New York.
   1. Public health.   I. Title.   II. Series.
RA431.H5   1977   614.4'4   76-40630
ISBN 0-405-09823-5

THE NEW PUBLIC HEALTH

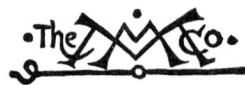

THE MACMILLAN COMPANY
NEW YORK · BOSTON · CHICAGO · DALLAS
ATLANTA · SAN FRANCISCO

MACMILLAN & CO., Limited
LONDON · BOMBAY · CALCUTTA
MELBOURNE

THE MACMILLAN CO. OF CANADA, Ltd.
TORONTO

The New Public Health

BY

HIBBERT WINSLOW HILL,
M. B., M. D., D. P. H.

Late Director, Division of Epidemiology, Minnesota State Board of Health, and later Executive Secretary, Minnesota Public Health Association, now Director, Institute of Public Health; and M. O. H., of London, Canada; Professor of Public Health, Western University.

New York
THE MACMILLAN COMPANY
1916

All rights reserved

COPYRIGHT, 1916,
BY THE MACMILLAN COMPANY.

Set up and electrotyped. Published February, 1916.

Norwood Press:
Berwick & Smith Co., Norwood, Mass., U.S.A.

PREFACE

THE conceptions of health, public and private, held by our ancestors and, until very lately, by ourselves, have undergone gradual revision, not to say revolution, in the last twenty years; changing most radically perhaps in the last ten. The Minnesota State Board of Health in 1911 designated the writer, then in charge of the Division of Epidemiology of that Board, to present the modern conceptions to the medical profession and to the public. A series of articles, which appeared monthly during 1912 in the *Journal-Lancet* of Minneapolis, was the outcome. These articles were furnished by the *Journal-Lancet* to 1,100 newspapers in the United States, and, during the latter half of the series, to fifty newspapers in Canada. Finally they were reprinted in book form at the end of the year. So cordial was their reception, that a revision and expansion of the articles thus first issued has been undertaken here.

The writer, in expressing his great personal debt to the State Board of Health of Minnesota for making possible this beginning and to the Board of Governors of the Institute of Public Health of London for its liberal support and continuation, would mention particularly Dr. W. A. Jones and Dr. H. M. Bracken, re-

PREFACE

spectively president and secretary of the Minnesota State Board of Health, Drs. B. M. Merrill and C. F. More, members of the Censorship Committee of that Board, and Mr. W. L. Klein, publisher of the *Journal-Lancet,* for their advice, deep personal interest, and cordial co-operation. To Dr. F. F. Wesbrook, now President of the University of British Columbia, then Director of the Minnesota State Board of Health Laboratories, to Dr. A. J. Chesley, then a colleague, now the writer's successor in the Division of Epidemiology, to Professor F. H. Bass, ex-Director of the Division of Sanitary Engineering of the Minnesota State Board of Health, to Mr. Christopher Easton, at one time Secretary of the Minnesota Anti-Tuberculosis Association, to Dr. J. P. Sedgwick of the Medical Department of the University of Minnesota, and to Professor S. Quigley of the Department of Pedagogy of the same University, the writer acknowledges with pleasure most friendly and valuable consultation on the more technical portions.

It is not possible to list all who have aided the writer directly or indirectly in this work; still less possible would it be to attempt to list those whose appreciation and good wishes made the work a pleasure. But it would be unseemly to omit reference to one other, who was unconnected with the official family either in Minnesota or in London. The great reconstructing force in Public Health has been bacteriology, but the application of the laboriously sought out and, to Public Health

PREFACE

principles, in general, often barren, work of the Bacteriologist, must be acknowledged as due to an administrator of keen insight and logical mind, Dr. Chas. V. Chapin of Providence, whose " Sources and Modes of Infection " marks the real beginning of scientific public health in America.

That this book may further aid in giving to all who read it a definite view of the chief problems of public health, and of their chief solutions, is the aim of the writer; that it may prove a satisfaction to many friends, his hope.

CONTENTS

CHAPTER		PAGE
I	DEFINITIONS	1
	SUMMARY	5
II	THE OLD PRINCIPLES AND THE NEW	7
	THE REVOLUTION	7
	THE OLD TEACHINGS	9
	THE NEW IDEAS	12
	ENVIRONMENT	14
III	INFECTIOUS DISEASES	17
	FACTS	17
	(a) SOURCES OF INFECTIOUS DISEASES	21
	(b) ROUTES OF INFECTIOUS DISEASES	23
	(c) CONTROL OF INFECTIOUS DISEASES	24
IV	WHY DO ANYTHING?	26
	HOW BIG A PROBLEM IS IT?	27
	WHO KEEPS THE INFECTIOUS DISEASE GOING?	28
	WHY AND HOW ARE WOMEN RESPONSIBLE?	29
	PRESENT ATTEMPTS	29
	RADICAL CHANGES IN SOCIAL CONDITIONS THE REAL SOLUTION	30
V	NON-INFECTIOUS DISEASES	33
	SPECULATIONS	33
	PHYSICAL PERFECTION	35
	THE GENERAL PROBLEM	36
	THE PRESENT SITUATION	39
	IMMEDIATE POSSIBILITIES	42
	EDUCATION	45

CONTENTS

CHAPTER		PAGE
	MEDICAL SUPERVISION OF SCHOOLS	48
	SUMMARY	50
VI	EDUCATIONAL MECHANISM	53
	SUMMARY	61
VII	THE OLD PRACTICE AND THE NEW	63
	EPIDEMIOLOGY	63
	COMPARATIVE METHODS	65
	THE NEW EMERGENCY EPIDEMIOLOGY	69
	STOPPING A "PRIMARY" EPIDEMIC	71
	STOPPING "SECONDARY" OUTBREAKS	73
	FINDING THE UNKNOWN CASES	75
	SUMMARY	77
VIII	THE NEWEST PRACTICE	79
	CONCURRENT EPIDEMIOLOGY	79
	FUTURE APPLICATIONS	84
	CHIEF INFECTIOUS DISEASES, CLASSIFIED BY ROUTES	88
	THE NEW PROGRAM	91
IX	INDIVIDUAL DEFENSE	95
	PUBLIC DEFENSE AND PRIVATE	95
	THE PREVENTABILITY OF THE "PREVENTABLE" DISEASES	96
	"DODGING INFECTION"	100
	CONTACT-INFECTION	101
	PLACARD FOR SCHOOLS	107
	SUMMARY	112
X	COMMUNITY DEFENSE	114
	THE PUBLIC HEALTH ENGINEER	114
	SUMMARY	122
XI	COMMUNITY DEFENSE	124
	THE PUBLIC HEALTH LABORATORY	124
	SUMMARY	131

CONTENTS

CHAPTER		PAGE
XII	COMMUNITY DEFENSE	133
	THE PUBLIC HEALTH STATISTICIAN	133
	STATISTICS AS THEY WILL BE	134
	STATISTICS AS THEY ARE	138
	SUMMARY	147
XIII	ADMINISTRATION	148
	SUMMARY	156
XIV	COMMUNITY DEFENSE APPLIED	158
	TUBERCULOSIS IN GENERAL	158
	HUMAN TUBERCULOSIS	159
	THE ABOLITION OF CATTLE TUBERCULOSIS FROM THE HUMAN	163
	THE ABOLITION OF HUMAN TUBERCULOSIS	163
	SUMMARY	170
XV	THE CONTROL OF DIPHTHERIA, SCARLET FEVER AND MEASLES	173
	SUMMARY	176
XVI	VENEREAL DISEASES	178
XVII	THE CONCLUSION OF THE WHOLE MATTER	182
	THE DOING OF IT	182
	THE CHIEF OBJECTIONS	185
	POPULAR FALLACIES	189
	NEW FASHIONED QUARANTINE	190
	SUMMARY	192
	APPENDIX I. CONDENSED DATA ON INFECTIOUS DISEASES	195
	APPENDIX II. SYLLABUS OF PUBLIC HEALTH TEACHING	197

THE NEW PUBLIC HEALTH

CHAPTER I

DEFINITIONS

PUBLIC HEALTH is a term which includes all knowledge and all measures tending to (a) foster health or (b) to prevent disease.

These two objects are far from identical. True, certain personal measures to promote health, classed under hygiene, i.e., proper care and cultivation of, say, the muscles, necessarily also avoids those " diseases," which may result from neglect or misuse of those muscles; incidentally, perhaps, of other parts of the body also. To care for properly and develop sight to its highest efficiency necessarily includes eliminating the train of evils connected with eye strain. But such cultivation of the body forces to secure high efficiency will not and cannot prevent those accidents or diseases which originate from outside sources. A bullet will travel equally as far through the soldier who is physically perfect as through him who is a physical wreck.

Public Health may be divided into Hygiene and Sanitation. Hygiene deals with the individual and his physical perfection. The causes and sources of those diseases which come from the outside, from the surroundings of the individual, are dealt with under the term Sanitation. Just as Hygiene deals with measures which (a) promote health and, some of them (b) prevent disease, so Sanitation also presents two subdivisions, the measures, dealing with surroundings, which intrinsically (a) promote health or (b) prevent disease. Thus, proper ventilation, while securing the best available conditions for the body so far as atmospheric surroundings are concerned, necessarily eliminates those " diseases " which might arise from the reaction of the body to " poor ventilation," and so far Sanitation and Hygiene are intimately interdependent. But good ventilation, although invaluable to the general welfare and efficiency of the body, has no necessary relation to the elimination of certain outside injurious forces, such as lead poisoning or alcoholism or accidents or invasions of the body by micro-organisms. Each of these must be met by specific measures, adapted to the elimination of the particular factor involved. Moreover, such specific measures will eliminate the specific trouble, whether such general physical efficiency and high health as may be secured through good ventilation be secured or not.

The greatest advance made of recent years in public health is the generalization from such facts, long known in detail, that measures promoting bodily health and efficiency do not necessarily eliminate those ex-

DEFINITIONS

ternal and insidious factors of disease by invasion from without, particularly of the invaders which produce the infectious diseases.

A third relationship, long believed and taught as existing between the measures for promoting health and those for eliminating disease, is fast losing its alleged importance. This belief is that which regards high health as not indeed abolishing infection, but as conferring an immunity against infectious diseases. It is beginning to be recognized that as " good ventilation " does not eliminate " eye strain," as good lighting does not correct " poor ventilation," so all through hygiene and sanitation specific troubles must be met by specific measures directed specifically against the real specific cause of that trouble. Taught for, lo these many years, that general cleanliness is a protection against disease, we are beginning to realize that only a specific cleanliness, that which actually eliminates disease germs, is of real value for this purpose; taught also that general high health protects against disease, we are beginning to understand that the only form of bodily condition which secures this end is the possession by the body of a specific protection against each specific disease.[1] Even should we admit that perfect health may theoretically

---

[1] It is far from certain that the process of securing such specific immunity *through an attack of the disease in question* does not involve permanent damage to the body incompatible with the subsequent attainment of the highest physical perfection.

prevent the inroads of smallpox or typhoid fever or pneumonia or colds, we would also have to admit that such high health is very readily upset, by a chill, a missed dinner, a day's overwork, a temporary indigestion; and since this is so, that the protection against infection afforded by such high health, if it exist at all, is too vague and uncertain, too subject to sudden alterations and even complete loss, to be worthy serious consideration as a real factor in the control of disease, in ordinary life. The value of high health, of hygiene, lies in the physical efficiency and bodily comfort which it bestows; in the sense of well being, in the energy, alertness and keenness which result from it. That it does not protect against infection, that it actually indirectly contributes to infection from the very fact that the energy and alertness it bestows take its possessor out where infection lies awaiting him, does not lessen its real value, but only makes the removal of the infection itself an even more important duty to the race. The man of "torpid liver" and bleary eye, the muscular wreck, lacks that vigor and aggressiveness which carry the possessor of high health out into the busy haunts of men and women; and to the extent that he escapes contact with his fellows, he tends to escape infection, just as the invalided soldier escapes the effects of bullets by not encountering them.

To hold that weaklings only, or principally, suffer from diseases of this nature is to hold a view which represents a complete reversal of the facts; indeed, if

DEFINITIONS

this view were true, infectious diseases would long since have weeded out all such weaklings and left a race of physically perfect giants, free from all diseases because of their exceeding physical perfection; whereas exactly the contrary is true, and we hear the cry everywhere that physical degeneracy is the bane of modern citizenship. Scarcely one-fifth of the young men examined for the U. S. army meet the much modified army requirements as to physique; moreover, that selected fifth, disciplined, exercised, fed and cared for at the highest level of hygiene that we know succumbs to infections quite as easily as their rejected brothers; and modern armies find high health and physical development so little a protection against these infections that every new specific, like vaccination, is seized upon eagerly to take its alleged place. Surely it is time to cease misleading the public and ourselves with a will-o'-the-wisp since the very teachers that lend their weight to the doctrine find in practice that no high health they can compass for their trained armies protects those armies in any adequate sense.

SUMMARY

Modern Public Health recognizes that health means much more than the mere absence of disease; and under Hygiene classes all measures to secure the best internal workings of the human frame to keep it at its best; thus eliminating the internal poisonings, and the results of deprivations and excesses which produce certain diseases or disabilities. But it recognizes further that surroundings, through direct action on the body, perfect or imperfect, may injure or destroy the best just as the worst; and under Sanitation, strives to provide surroundings which may eliminate external conditions leading to disease or injury.

The chief advance of recent years is that which recognizes the specificity of cause and effect, both in Hygiene and in Sanitation; and meets each separate source or cause of each such trouble with a specific measure to prevent it.

Against the visible outside causes of disease, those causes which can be seen and recognized by every one, (the chemical poisons, accidents, etc.), the weapons are education and elimination or proper handling of those causes, if they cannot be eliminated.

Against the invisible and, to the general public, unrecognizable causes which produce the infectious diseases, the warfare must necessarily be directed to their elimination, under such preliminary education as will permit the establishment of the necessary mechanisms.

CHAPTER II

THE OLD PRINCIPLES AND THE NEW

THE REVOLUTION

THE statement that there is a " New Public Health " may shock those who, although familiar with recent changes in scientific thought, yet have not fully realized what those changes mean; but the shock will be far greater to those who have not appreciated that changes were going on.

The purpose of the writer is to formulate for both groups, the unconscious progressive and the unconscious conservative, a brief statement of the essential principles of modern professional public health work relating to the prevention of disease. To those who may feel skeptical as to the fairness of this exposition, the writings of Chapin, the great American pioneer of modern public health, of E. O. Jordan, and of M. N. Baker, may be offered as bearing directly upon these questions, while the whole of modern technical public-health literature may be offered as indirect evidence. Since the infectious diseases constitute the chief as well as the best understood group of preventable diseases or causes of death and disability, the infectious diseases are here chiefly discussed.

The old principles have merged gradually into the new, in keeping with the experiments, observations, and conclusions of many investigators in many individual sciences related to general public health. Within professional public-health circles, bacteriology, clinical observation, and mathematics have furnished most of the reconstruction. The bacteriologist, the epidemiologist, and the vital statistician, sometimes working together, more often alone, in the dark and even at cross purposes, have nevertheless all reached the same point, and to-day each finds his co-workers beside him. Much of the work done has consisted in clearing away the fallacies built up by tradition, but construction-work has gone on also, and it is now possible to formulate the results.

The essential change is this: The old public health was concerned with the environment; the new is concerned with the individual. The old sought the sources of infectious disease in the surroundings of man; the new finds them in man himself.

The old public health sought these sources in the air, in the water, in the earth, in the climate and topography of localities, in the temperature of soils at four and six feet deep, in the rise and fall of ground-waters; it failed because it sought them, very painstakingly and exhaustively, it is true, in every place and in every thing *where they were not*.

The new public health seeks these sources — and finds them — amongst those infective persons (or animals) whose excreta or other constituents or body contents enter the bodies of other persons.

The old public health failed to find the sources of infection; it also failed in most instances to find the routes of transmission. It is true that public water-supplies were detected as at times transmitting infection; but milk was hardly suspected twenty years ago; flies (and other insects), suggested in 1887,[1] were not seriously considered until the Spanish-American war; mouth-spray [2] and hands have been only recently recognized as important. On the other hand, dirty clothes, bad smells, damp cellars, leaky plumbing, dust, foul air, rank vegetation, swamps, stagnant pools, certain soils, smoke, garbage, manure, dead animals, in fact everything physically, sensorially, esthetically, or psychically objectionable, were lumped together as "unsanitary" without much distinction of "source" or "route," and were regarded as a sort of general "cause of disease" to be condemned wherever found, "for fear of epidemics."

THE OLD TEACHINGS

It was taught that infectious diseases "generated" in the foul, ill-smelling, unventilated, sunless hovels of the slums. In the vogue of those days, " the slum-dwellers

[1] Wm. H. Welch: Address at the Annual Meeting of the Medical and Chirurgical Faculty of Maryland 1887, quoted in *Sewage and Local Drainage.*— Waring, 1889.

[2] By this is meant the fine droplets thrown out from the mouth in speaking, singing, laughing, sneezing, coughing, etc.

live like pigs, and thereby invoke the coming of smallpox, scarlet fever, typhoid fever, diphtheria." When these diseases invaded the home of the well-to-do, where this explanation was not seemly, a pinhole leak in some plumbing fixture accounted amply for diphtheria; rotten potatoes, forgotten in a dark corner of the cellar, for typhoid fever; scarlet fever was traced to a letter bearing "scales" from a friend who had had the disease months before; smallpox to unpacking books used by a patient a quarter of a century previously; manure piles gave rise to cholera; and dampness to malaria, which was not recognized as transmissible at all. Yellow fever originated in impure water and was directly transmitted from person to person — a typical example of intense direct contagion; tuberculosis was non-infectious and hereditary; bubonic plague was banished from the Egyptian Cairo "simply by improving the ventilation of the city" (!)[3]

Remedial and preventive measures, based on such beliefs in the omnipotence of environment, naturally sought to remodel the lives and immediate home surroundings of the whole population to conform with a vast array of alleged "sanitary laws of health." Yet he who seeks for a scientific demonstration of the relations existing between disobedience of these "sanitary laws" on the one hand, and the incidence of disease and death on the other, will find only a "twilight zone"

[3] Parke's *Hygiene*, 1891; eighth edition. This was a standard work of twenty-five years ago.

OLD PRINCIPLES AND NEW

in which move vague shadows of traditional fear, shadows which, on probing, fade mistily away.[4]

While admitting freely that almost any item of an environment may act as a route of infection, at odd times, or under peculiar conditions, the New Public Health is not worried by elaborate theoretical possibilities, but concerns itself earnestly with practical probabilities. The occasional, unusual, bizarre routes of infection in the 1 per cent. of cases, do not distract its attention from the usual, practically constant, simple, ordinary routes concerned in the 99 per cent. Its main postulate is that the routes of infection are simply the routes of infected bodily discharges, which, again, are identical with the routes of ordinary uninfected discharges in ordinary life; and that if the 99 per cent. of commonplace cases are prevented, the 1 per cent. will not occur at all. Too often attention has been riveted on extreme precautions to avoid the 1 per cent., and no precautions worthy of the name have been directed to avoidance of the 99 per cent.

The old style " sanitary inspector " was expected to, and usually did, " condemn " everything in sight, from the garbage pail at the back door to the plumbing in the bath-room. But disease continued, because he was condemning, as a rule, so far as health was concerned, things largely " incompetent, irrelevant and immaterial." What availed it that the garbage-pail was emptied every day or a vent-pipe placed on the bath-

[4] See *Journal-Lancet* of July 15, 1914.

water waste-trap, if the milkman delivered scarlet-fever-infected milk at the door, or an unrecognized case of measles sat next the children at school?

The wooden knight of *Alice in Wonderland* who carried a mouse trap on horseback because mice *might* some day infest his horse, while riding so badly that he continually fell off on his head and was as continually in process of being restored to his saddle by kind friends, furnishes the most kindly yet realistic satire on prevailing public-health methods that could well be devised.

THE NEW IDEAS

The New Public Health sees in the garbage-pail merely a place where flies are fed and, possibly, bred. But the flies cannot carry infection *if infected discharges are not accessible to them.*

The Old regarded the garbage-pail as in itself and by itself intrinsically bad, disease-producing and deleterious to health. This, notwithstanding that employes in garbage-collection, garbage-destruction or garbage-rendering work average as healthy a body of men as any others of similar status.

"Defective plumbing," such a nightmare twenty years ago, has been conclusively shown to have nothing to do with disease-generation or disease-propagation whatever, unless perchance there be actual gross leakage of infected sewage. The employees connected with great sewage systems, even those continually employed

OLD PRINCIPLES AND NEW 13

in the great sewers of large cities, average well, like garbage workers, as to incidence of disease amongst them.

The unventilated front parlor could not produce tuberculosis in a hundred years; diphtheria does not develop from the family well despite many a well-meant tirade on its evils; and typhoid fever, in sand or clay areas, is but seldom properly traceable to that source, either. Stagnant or old, longstanding water, is to this day often considered responsible for typhoid, despite the definite knowledge that no system of purification of typhoid-infected water is more reliable than impounding, which is merely keeping it standing!

The modern public health man cares nothing, so far as restriction of disease and death is concerned, for the dirty back yard or the damp cellar in themselves, but only as they may enter into the transmission of infected discharges. Then, at once, they become of vital importance. The sanitary inspection of the modern sanitarian, so far as relates to infection, begins and usually ends with the search for (a) the infected individual; (b) the routes of spread of infection from that individual; (c) the routes of spread of the ordinary excreta of ordinary uninfected individuals to the mouths of their ordinary associates in ordinary life. These latter are sought for, not because of danger from such uninfected discharges, but rather because infected discharges, introduced into and following the same well-beaten paths, will necessarily reach the same mouths.

To locate all the infective persons and to guard all their discharges would be wholly sufficient and is the ultimate goal of modern preventive measures, but since this cannot always be done perfectly, it is well to guard also the routes which unlocated infection may take.

ENVIRONMENT

Has environment, then, nothing to do with infectious diseases? Environment acts in two ways: First, unequivocally and without reserve, such environments as permit or encourage or, still worse, necessitate the exchange of human excreta in ordinary life, contribute in the long run to the spread of disease since they insure a similar exchange of infected excreta so soon as the latter are introduced.[5] Let us take one environmental evil, overcrowding, as an example. Overcrowding, if combined with lack of discipline and order, and lack of facilities for washing, especially for the washing of hands, contributes to the spread of infectious diseases; but not in itself; nor at all, unless infection be introduced into the community. Then overcrowding, because it tends to insure exchange of human excreta, tends also to insure that the infection will spread rapidly and extensively. But overcrowding, if the overcrowded be disciplined, intelligent, and take proper precautions to avoid exchange of excreta, does not necessi-

[5] An excellent exposition of this effect of environment on the spread of disease is given by Chapin in the Report of the Providence Health Department for 1910.

tate the spread of infection, even if it be introduced. On the other hand, infection may spread, and frequently does, without overcrowding, if the essential factor of such spread exist, i.e., the transmission of infected excreta.

Second. Environments that are bad from a physiological standpoint (bad for the body, regarded as a delicate biological machine) are often held to act in spreading infection indirectly by " depressing vitality " to an extent which makes infection, if received, more likely to develop (and if it develop, more successful in injuring the body). It must be said, however, that the evidence on this point, except perhaps that relating to tuberculosis and pneumonia, is very slight. It is a debatable question whether or not overcrowding " depresses vitality " in the direction of increasing susceptibility to infectious diseases, whatever its effect may be in encouraging " general debility." It is a very debatable question whether or not " poor ventilation," to which the effects of overcrowding are often attributed, can or does " depress vitality " in the direction of lessening resistance to infectious diseases, whatever bad effects it may have on mental vigor or physical activity. It is true that there is evidence that such environments as lead to extremes (beyond the limits of compensatory adjustments by the body forces) of mal-nutrition, of temperature, of fatigue, and of alcoholism, probably may have an effect in insuring the development of infection, which under better conditions might be negatived by the body forces. Especially may these forms of bad physiological environment be influential when the dose of infection is small, infrequent, or low in virulence, for it is conceivable that under good environment the body might "throw them off more readily." But starvation, unsuitable temperature, fatigue, alcoholism, alone or together, cannot induce infection, nor will the converse conditions, alone or together, offset the effects of infection when the dose is large or frequently repeated or of high virulence.

CHAPTER III

INFECTIOUS DISEASES

FACTS

It would appear, then, that environment as affecting bodily functions has little to do directly with the incidence of most of the specific infections,[1] notwithstanding that nutrition, temperature, fatigue, and alcoholism are generally credited with some effect, especially in pneumonia and tuberculosis.

Damp, cold, and fatigue perhaps precipitate the pneumonias, although the relation is not clear, and of course no such effect is observed unless one of the infective agents be present. The environments if there be such at all, that precipitate tuberculosis constitute a problem as yet unsolved. Very much is widely believed, and even more is freely taught, concerning this subject, but the evidence is tangled and often contra-

[1] The terms *contagious* and *infectious* were formerly carefully used and carefully distinguished. Modern writers, however, fail to find any useful or basic significance in " contagious " as contrasted with " infectious." Hektoen, in Osler's *Modern Medicine*, discards " contagious " and " contagion " entirely.

In these articles " infectious " is used to mean " transmissible " or " communicable."

dictory. "Poor ventilation," dust, dampness, etc., have all been accused, but very little has been proved concerning the real factors actually at work or their mode of operation. In the other infectious diseases the effects even of extremes of the above factors are but rarely definitely recognizable.

Smallpox is contracted or escaped in exact ratio to the degree of exposure acting in opposition to the degree of specific immunity. No other known environmental factor, even acute alcoholism, is recognized as influential.

One thing, and one thing only, is absolutely established, namely, that tuberculosis, microbic pneumonia, and the other infectious diseases will develop under almost any circumstances if the dose of infection be large enough, virulent enough, or sufficiently repeated. Tuberculosis, microbic pneumonia, and the other infectious diseases will not develop under any circumstances without such infection.

Hence it must be evident that the *sine qua non* of all infectious diseases are their respective agents, and that, since the chief sources (infective persons) of these are known, the most logical efforts are those which concentrate on the prevention of the dissemination of these agents from these sources.

This is tenable, not only in theory, but in practice, and presents an infinitely simpler administrative problem than that presented by the older hypotheses,— not only in the "minor" infectious diseases, where these

INFECTIOUS DISEASES

principles have been practically accepted by all, but even in tuberculosis itself.

Thus, if " general environment " be the great factor in tuberculosis, the hundred million people of these United States must have each his or her own individual environment brought up to and kept at some standard-level designed to maintain each individual in his or her own alleged " highest state of health."

If, however, the infectiveness of the disease be the great factor, only 200,000 people (the actively infective cases) need this supervision in the United States, and they need it, not for the improvement of their " general environment," but *merely to prevent them from infecting others.* This problem, even numerically, is but one five-hundredth the magnitude of the other. Consider the utterly impracticable expense and difficulty of the attempt to insure only the four quoted factors,— good food, proper temperatures, temperance, and repose,— to one hundred million people (to say nothing of the other " factors of safety " called for by those who lay chief emphasis on control of environment, i.e., abolition of foul air, smoke, dust, damp cellars, bad smells, dirty back yards, etc.), and contrast with this the expense of supervision of two hundred thousand people *merely to the extent of confining their infective discharges to themselves.*

Further consider that the same official mechanism which could control the tuberculous could also handle with but slight expansion the infectious persons needing supervision for the prevention of all the other infectious diseases, except the venereal, as well as the infective tuberculous. Remember also that improvement of the "general environment," allowing that its effective achievement were conceivable, could not be expected to have any noteworthy effect on most of these other infectious diseases, even though it had some on tuberculosis.

Need any more be said to indicate the superiority of the new principles, as practical business propositions, over the old?

The stumbling-block is that the general public still believes the teachings of twenty years ago concerning environment. These teachings were a mixture of the "old-wives fables" of the prebacterial age, with the early incongruities and half-truths of the new "theory" of bacteriology.

Bacteriology is now an old-established science; but despite the fact that it has changed public-health work even more than it has changed medicine or surgery,— and both of these it has completely revolutionized,— the public still clings to the belief that public health is a curious profession, absorbedly interested in cutting weeds in vacant lots ("to prevent epidemics"), in burying dead animals and suppressing noisome odors ("to prevent epidemics"); in inspecting plumbing and collecting garbage ("to prevent epidemics"). The "good" health officer according to the popular standard, still too prevalent, is he who keeps the streets clean

INFECTIOUS DISEASES

and the back alleys neat, who falls into a rapture over a newly whitewashed outhouse and into a rampage if a pile of old bones is found under the cellar steps. Yet many of those who know better let these ideas alone, or even acquiesce in them, "to save trouble." Nevertheless it is expected that the thus carefully uneducated, or miseducated, public opinion will demand up-to-date action! Is it any wonder that the public insists on thinking, acting, and legislating to suit the theories of twenty years ago instead of the scientific knowledge of to-day?

Brief formulations of intricate principles are often misleading, incomplete, or fallacious; yet the temptation to formulate the new principles briefly is strong, because their intelligent presentation to the public is so vital. Such formulation is attempted here.

a. *Sources of Infectious Diseases*

1. Infectious diseases are infectious because they are due to the growth, in the body, of minute animal or vegetable forms (germs), the transmissibility of these germs from body to body being the sole explanation why these diseases are "catching."

2. Wherever in the body the germs develop, they leave it chiefly in the discharges, or by routes of the discharges, of the nose and throat, bladder, or bowel, i.e., from the main orifices of the body.[2]

---

[2] This applies to all the ordinary infectious diseases in this zone. Smallpox, leprosy, syphilis, and some forms of tubercu-

3. The discharges infect another person practically only when that person takes the discharges, in some form, into the mouth or nose, except in trachoma and the venereal diseases.[3]

4. Outside the body, disease germs do not multiply in nature, except perhaps rarely, and very temporarily, in milk, water, or similar fluids. In general, even typhoid bacilli disappear from water supplies within two weeks, without evident multiplication. If introduced into milk, most infectious-disease germs die out as the milk becomes acid, generally in a day or two. Infectious-disease germs are rarely found in garbage, and they quickly die out if deliberately added. Practical modern public health recognizes therefore that the bulk of most of the infectious diseases are derived directly, or almost directly, from infected persons, not much from infected things, except recently infected water, milk, food, and flies. The danger from the general environment of an infected person is therefore small. The *things* in his neighborhood need little consideration, except those very immediately about him and directly infected by his discharges, such as bedclothes, personal clothes, towels, eating utensils, and

losis are transferable from skin lesions at times. Certain tropical diseases are transmitted by insects tapping the blood-stream, etc. Probably all infections can be conveyed, as anthrax and tetanus usually are, directly by inoculation. But these paths are so rare as to be negligible in ordinary life here.

[3] "Infection is transmitted from an orifice of the infector to an orifice of the infectee."

INFECTIOUS DISEASES

other material objects that may receive, and retain for a time, fresh moist discharges. If attention be efficiently directed to infected persons and their discharges, the general surroundings may be safely ignored, except in the rarest instances. Disinfection of premises recently occupied by infectious persons (terminal disinfection), a few years ago considered on theoretical grounds as one of the chief weapons against disease, has, on practical investigation been very largely abandoned except in tuberculosis, where practical investigation shows that it is of some value, if the premises are to be used within a month or so.

b. *Routes of Infectious Diseases*

5. The routes by which the discharges of the sick person pass to the well person are exactly those by which the same discharges pass from the well person to the well person in ordinary life; for nose and mouth discharges the routes are mouth-spray, and sputum conveyed through direct contact (as in kissing, etc.), and by the hands; for bowel and bladder discharges, the hands chiefly; and for all discharges, the things infected by them directly or through the hands, especially those things which then go to the mouth or touch things which go to the mouth, as food, water, eating utensils, towels, pipes, etc., etc. Flies also furnish an effective route, especially from feces to food. Water supplies are peculiar, because bowel and bladder discharges *en masse,* in the form of sewage, often enter them di-

rectly, at times being deliberately poured into them from city sewers.

6. The relative importance of these various routes in the carriage of infection varies much. The amount and freshness of the discharges, the number and virulence of the germs they contain, the size and frequency of the dose, and the number of susceptible persons who are dosed, must always be considered. Almost all the ordinary infectious-disease germs die out quickly on exposure to direct sunlight, and fairly rapidly in diffuse sunlight. When mucus, feces, and urine are thoroughly dried on furniture, door-knobs, etc., they are not readily removed again without moisture and friction, and when so removed the disease germs in them are likely to be dead or greatly reduced in recuperative power because of the drying. Hence, as a rule, *things* succeed in conveying infection only somewhat directly from the infector to the infectee, and practically only during the limited period when the germs are still fresh and moist.

c. *Control of Infectious Diseases*

7. These new principles place at the head of official public health activities, the search for and supervision of infected persons, and the control of the infected discharges, for the purpose of excluding them from mouths, and therefore also from food and drink. Prompt intelligent disinfection of all the excreta *immediately after their discharge from the body* (concurrent

INFECTIOUS DISEASES

disinfection), is the best weapon in the supervision of infected persons. Isolation of the infected person is the next best, and is more universally practicable, because immediate intelligent disinfection of discharges can rarely be secured outside of the very best hospitals for contagious disease. The search for and supervision of mild, early, convalescing, unrecognized, and concealed cases and carriers, as well as of frank cases, is necessarily an essential item in the scheme.

8. The modern public-health department requires experts, but not experts in municipal house-keeping, in street-cleaning, garbage-disposal, smoke-prevention, etc. Its experts are the vital statistician, the epidemiologist, the laboratory man, and the sanitary engineer, the latter dealing chiefly with the broad questions of water-supply and sewage-disposal.

CHAPTER IV

WHY DO ANYTHING?

It has been well said that the day of the priest in public health has passed: to-day is the day of the doctor; but I think that to-morrow will be the day of the business man, the man of large affairs; and it is to him this chapter is addressed.

Until such time as poverty is abolished, or the State takes charge of children, the majority of the women of the race must continue to rear the majority of the children of the race inadequately, in homes too small, without facilities, doing for them somehow, individually and alone, that which three women could hardly do well, working together.

This is not wholly a slum problem nor is it a problem of the rich. Numerically the race is chiefly middle class, neither rich nor extremely poor, judged by ordinary standards. This is the problem of the family with an income below $3,000, i.e., it is the problem of the race proper, and it is the old problem of the premosaic Hebrew — how to make bricks without straw — alas, often without knowing how to make bricks at all!

The problem as a whole involves food, clothing, proper physical development, morals, education, amusement, discipline, and citizenship. But the public hygienist has *as yet* but indirect concern with these. The public hygienist — the " board of health man "— *as yet* concerns himself chiefly and by general expectation and consent, with the grosser, more imminent, more spectacular, more immediately tragic, problems of disease and death, and chiefly with only one group of these, the infectious diseases. However much in ordinary life overcrowding, lack of facilities and overburdening of mothers may render unavailing even the tears and ageing, the back-ache, heart-ache, crooked fingers and wrinkled faces of mothers striving for their young, ten times over is the effect of these seen when disease enters the family, adding its burdens, its sorrows, its disabilities and its deaths.

Once more, remember this is not in the slums alone, nor, numerically, chiefly there. It is found in city and country, village and town, everywhere, the overburdening of mothers, in ordinary life, added to ten times over when disease springs up.

HOW BIG A PROBLEM IS IT?

Call the population of the United States 100,000,000. Remember that, sooner or later, every member of each generation suffers from at least one infectious disease, often from two, three or four, and it is clear that every generation suffers anywhere from 100,000,000 to 300,-000,000 attacks of infections. Each generation pays out at least ten billions of dollars for this running of the gauntlet, not to speak of the disability and death of those who run it unsuccessfully. Tuberculosis, diphtheria, summer diarrhea, scarlet fever, measles, typhoid fever, whooping cough, chickenpox, to name only some of those best known to the laity, how much sorrow, distress, poverty, how much "making of none avail" of mothers' hopes and prayers and wearing effort have these caused! Yet so common are they that "children's diseases" are looked upon as a necessary stage, almost a joke. Indeed some people deliberately expose their children to them, "to have it over with"! Yet who bears the burden, the sleepless nights, the extra work, the hope deferred?

Ninety-five per cent. of the infectious diseases are nursed at home by mothers. Next to the children themselves the ones who suffer most are mothers.

WHO KEEPS THE INFECTIOUS DISEASE GOING?

Once more the answer is — and most emphatically — women in general, but chiefly after all the mother. To be sure there is every excuse for the mother,— overwork, overcrowding, lack of facilities, above all ignorance and misdirected training, "misinformation piled on lack of any." But with all the perfectly good apologies stated and all the excellent good-will and effort counted in, the fact itself remains, that mothers propagate and keep alive and spread the infectious diseases of children more than any other one body of people, and that while conditions remain as they are they

WHY DO ANYTHING? 29

must learn the "rules of the game" and follow them, for no amount of coaching or effort from the sidelines can do more than help.

WHY AND HOW ARE WOMEN RESPONSIBLE?

Because mothers are doing the work — women in general, but chiefly mothers. The farmer is responsible (apart from flood, drought, storm or other "acts of God") for whatever happens to the crop from seed to market. Women in general — but chiefly mothers — are the "raisers" and "crop-handlers" of the largest, most valuable, most expensive and most difficult crop in the country. What happens to this crop between birth and sixteen years of age is, chiefly, what women do to it, or at least do not prevent. For the first 5,000 days of the years of the life of each generation, the race is fed, dressed, undressed, washed, combed, cuddled, kissed, praised, blamed, led, driven, coaxed, taught, spanked, bossed and otherwise "brought up" by women — women mothers at home, women teachers at school. It is chiefly during this time of tutelage and supervision by women that children receive their infections; it is during this time that the race runs its gauntlet, dances its little dance with death — and pays ten billions for it.

PRESENT ATTEMPTS

To teach women, girls, prospective mothers, that they may practice in their households, and in turn teach their children to war on invisible germ-foes is one of the functions of public health bacteriology. Only in the public schools can it be taught with emphasis, weight and uniformity enough to impress the masses. Only if taught in the grades can it be counted upon to reach the masses. Less than 1 per cent. of the population reach the university, only 10 per cent. reach the high schools. The great mass of the mothers of the coming generation, of the whole race, the mothers of more than their average of children, are receiving grade school education only. Need more be said?

The infectious diseases in general radiate from and are kept going by women. Women must learn to break up, divert, stop in some manner — in every manner — the exchange of infected discharges amongst children at school and amidst families at home if infectious diseases are to be abolished or abated under present conditions. The needful information, beliefs, technique and habits cannot be had or established except by studying the basic principles of public health, and this must be taught in the grades of the public schools if it is to reach those who most need it.

RADICAL CHANGES IN SOCIAL CONDITIONS THE REAL SOLUTION

If (as cannot be) every girl now at grade school could be thoroughly taught all that a trained nurse knows, theory and practice, the best to be hoped is that, be-

WHY DO ANYTHING? 31

coming a mother, ten to twenty years hence, she may remember enough to care for, if she have the facilities, the first case of infection in her household without permitting its spread to the other members or to outsiders. Alas, not one-third of the girls will remember, not one-tenth will have the facilities. Above all what shall be done in that intervening ten to twenty years? Lectures, writings, sermons, appeals to mothers' clubs, university extensions, moving pictures, all the publicity that can be had or hoped for, will not suffice to teach technique to the mothers now in possession of the coming generation. Nor once more, if it taught them, would it provide the facilities needed. Economic conditions must change and change specifically to aid the mother if we are to gain at all. Also, the prevention of disease must engage the serious attention of governments — the *prevention* of disease, not the talking about it or the looking wise over it, or the making of fine addresses on it, but *preventing* it. Such prevention *may* include a tremendous organization to prevent human discharges entering water supplies, milk supplies, food supplies; must involve watchfulness of hotels, restaurants, public institutions of all sorts — in short, of all public alimentary utilities, with all their off-shoots and side issues wherever found. It *must* include, as its chief and most efficient weapon, the finding of the sources of infection, and the prevention of spread of infection from those sources. This is peculiarly a governmental function, but the whole must be cooperative. The government must strike at the sources and at the public routes of infection. The woman must strike at the private routes. The man must support both methods for the sake of the women and children.

CHAPTER V

NON-INFECTIOUS DISEASES

SPECULATIONS

The previous chapters indicated that so far as the infectious diseases are concerned, the great public-health fallacy of the nineteenth century consisted in the devotion of nearly all the effort to man's surroundings; of almost none at all to man himself. We know now that the sources of infection are in man; that the routes of infection are the routes of man's discharges; and that the discharges are harmless until they enter man again. It is true that when the infective agents reach their goal the resistance of the individual, pitted against the injurious powers of the infective agents, decides whether or not actual disease develops. But this resistance of the individual is not to be measured by his surroundings: it is intrinsic in himself. Alterations of intrinsic resistance do, of course, constantly occur, but the factors of those alterations are not, as a rule, to be readily ascertained. We think that great extremes of malnutrition, temperature, and so forth may "depress" resistance. We have evidence that the smoke nuisance, poor ventilation, or smells from slaughter-houses do not. In brief, granted sufficient exposure to infectious disease, the susceptible individual will succumb, though he live in a palace; the immune individual will escape, though he dwell in the slums.[1]

The immunity may be natural — born with the individual — or acquired, but this is beside the question. Far more practically important is the fact that the immunity, natural or acquired, is specific. The individual may be wholly immune to one disease and ultra-susceptible to another; and such immunity has absolutely no relation to physique, robustness, or great vitality.

The outcome of the environmental doctrines was the binding of heavy burdens of routine administration concerning surroundings upon health departments. Results: garbage disposal, a polytechnic trade; street-cleaning, a scientific profession; plumbing, a fine art; and the supervision of infection, a dubious and usually a temporary " job," too often left to utter incompetents, or to those who, competent enough, are unable to devote any systematic energy and very little time to it.

We have pursued chimeras; pursued them in good faith of course, but chimeras none the less.

Suppose now that we admit our errors and give to

[1] Tuberculosis has long been held an exception to this rule. But tuberculosis was also held as (a) non-infectious and (b) hereditary, as well as (c) a result of certain surroundings. We have reversed (a); we have reversed (b); we already see good reasons to modify (c).

NON-INFECTIOUS DISEASES

the supervision of tuberculosis,[2] which we do understand, one-half the effort we have given to the supervision of ventilation, which we are only beginning to understand. Suppose, in brief, we really organize and really operate a real machine which really does reduce, even promises to abolish, the infectious diseases. Will it be a surrender of our birthrights for a mess of pottage if in devoting ourselves to the suppression of disease at first hand, we forego the chasing down of loose paper on the streets and the cleaning up of rubbish piles on vacant lots?

PHYSICAL PERFECTION

There are activities contributing to health beyond these limits, of course; and some of them are things that should be done at once without waiting for the complete suppression of disease. For example, every one knows that the bodily welfare of mankind does not by any means hinge wholly on the infectious diseases. True, the abolition of these diseases means also the abolition of their immediate sequelæ,— sometimes, as in measles, more harmful than the original attack,— and of their remote sequelæ, the permanently injured kidney and the permanently weakened lung. But even so, a full half of our medical diseases and much more than half of our surgical diseases would still remain; moreover, merely to remove disease is not to solve the whole

[2] To say nothing of syphilis, gonorrhea, summer diarrhea, and the rest.

problem of securing health in its true sense, i.e., the highest physical efficiency prolonged for the greatest period of time.

THE GENERAL PROBLEM

The chief of the many phases of disease and health are best shown by a parable:

As a new automobile is accompanied by detailed instructions for its care and operation, so the new small citizen should be accompanied by detailed instructions for *his* care and operation when he, a delicate and complicated machine, indeed, first appears on the scene. This knowledge is now accumulated by his parents chiefly from experience (which, remember, are *his* experiences) or by picking it up at random from the neighbors over the back-yard fence. To secure proper results, the instruction of the mother should precede the birth of the child; and the proper care of the child involves proper care of the mother before the child is born. Prenatal and postnatal care are almost equally important to the child, and the former is peculiarly valuable to the mother.

Again: As a new automobile is searched solicitously for missing or defective parts, to be solicitously and immediately made good before the machine is sent out to run against competitors on the highway, so the new small citizen should have at least his sight, his hearing, and his breathing tested before he begins the inevitable compulsory-education race against all comers on the pub-

NON-INFECTIOUS DISEASES

lic highway of the public schools. Pre-school supervision will soon antedate school supervision. Why should the child suffer for its first five years defects and disabilities which are to be systematically corrected in the sixth? But further: As the most initially perfect automobile, most skillfully run, will yet, as time goes on, meet accidents, develop internal disruptions, and require repairs, so the new small citizen, despite early care and early correction of defects, will need supervision and repair all through his life, at school and afterwards.

The parable must end here, for automobiles present no affections analogous to infectious diseases. This very fact, however, brings out more clearly the crucial distinction between man as a machine and man as a subject of infection. As a machine, he may be efficient or inefficient, well operated or ill operated, and this all quite apart from the existence of actual defect or disability. Contrariwise, as a machine he may suffer initial defects or encounter accidents or develop internal disruptions, all quite apart from his intrinsic efficiency or inefficiency and quite apart from the skill with which he is operated. But as a subject of infection, man is merely a soil more or less well suited to the growth of certain small plants, or animals.[3]

The most valuable production of the State is its citi-

[3] The fact that in their growth these little invaders from without "mess up the works" and make trouble, as much as would disruptions originating wholly from within, should not conceal the radical difference between the sources and causes of defects,

zens; and the State, properly conceived, exists only to insure life, liberty, and the pursuit of happiness to them. As the automobile maker insists, *for his own sake,* on (a) giving instructions and (b) correcting defects; so the State should, *for its own sake,* (a) instruct parents and (b) remedy children's defects, perhaps also the defects, disabilities, and diseases of adults. Certainly, every State should provide at least —

Education for parents in the personal hygiene of children, i.e., the care and operation of their children's bodies as machines; and education also for children in the physical care of themselves.

Supervision, not only for the mere detection, but also for the remedy, of initial defects; and should provide this early in life, the earlier the better, certainly not later than the beginning of the compulsory-education course.

Supervision of children, at least throughout school-life, for the detection, *and remedy,* of such defects, disabilities, or diseases as may develop during that period.[4]

Finally, the supervision of infectious diseases.

disabilities, and non-infectious diseases on the one hand, and of the infectious diseases on the other. The former may develop in any mechanism; the latter only in those mechanisms which furnish a suitable soil for the growth of the extraneous invaders. To prevent the former the machine must be well built and of the best stock, must be scrupulously watched for defects, must be constantly overhauled, and must be cared for and operated in the most skilful manner. To prevent the latter the mere exclusion of the invaders is all-sufficient.

[4] It is difficult to see strictly logical reasons why such super-

NON-INFECTIOUS DISEASES

THE PRESENT SITUATION

But of all these manifold duties of the State to the citizen, only one of those which can be clearly shown to bear directly on his bodily welfare has been, as yet, fully recognized — only one rests on definite precedent, authorization and organization; and that one is the supervision of infectious diseases. The personal hygiene of the citizen (*apart from the infectious diseases*), and the *remedy* (even, until lately, the mere *detection*) of his defects, disabilities, or non-infectious diseases, have been regarded (except in the case of the pauper, the criminal, or the insane) as of little or no interest to any one but himself. And this, notwithstanding that all his material surroundings, and all his relationships, business and social, have been of acknowledged interest to the State from time immemorial. The sanitation of environment has indeed had much attention; usually misdirected and almost always inefficient, so far as abolishing infections is concerned.

Why this negligence of the individual, with excessive, misguided, attention to his surroundings? First, because material surroundings are property, and property has always had precedence over persons in almost every relation; second, because, in the special relation to disease, the old public health taught that the citizen was a

vision should end with school-life. Germany and England are experimenting with the medical supervision of adults. Prenatal and postnatal supervision are already United States Federal projects. Minnesota is agitating pre-school supervision.

resultant of his surroundings; and even in the infectious diseases this fallacy ruled, as has been abundantly shown.

Of course, the State is concerned with man's surroundings and relationships. It must consider, plan for, and carry out, measures for his comfort, convenience, safety, pleasure, and happiness, as well as merely for his health. The State exists to do for its citizens co-operatively, hence economically and authoritatively, all those necessary things which the individual could do only by great sacrifices or perhaps not at all. But to believe that the securing to the individual of every possible advantage in all directions is the duty of the State, is not necessarily to believe that every item of this program should be carried out by health departments. To hand over to any one subdivision of the government control both of man and of his surroundings, would be to hand over to it all the functions of government. At once, subdivision of these activities would be necessary and these subdivisions would necessarily pattern after those of present governments. Hence such a "readjustment" would merely replace existing governments, not add to their existing efficiency.

The secret of successful organization is the parcelling out *along natural lines* of all the different activities which are to be co-ordinated to one great end. It is upon the shrewdness with which the subdivision into logical natural groups is done that the securing of smoothly-running co-ordination depends. Certainly,

NON-INFECTIOUS DISEASES

one most logical grand division of any government would be that which should deal with man apart from his surroundings; and one most logical subdivision of that unit should deal with his bodily welfare as distinct from his mental, moral, or other welfare.

Using the automobile parable for guidance, such a "Commission on Bodily Welfare" should deal with —

Item 1. The education of *every citizen* in personal hygiene.

Item 2. The supervision of *every citizen* for detection of defects, disabilities, and disease.

Item 3. The treatment of *every citizen* for all defects, disabilities, and diseases detected.

Item 4. Finally, that function to which the automobile analogy does not apply, i.e., the supervision of that small group of citizens, the infectious persons.

How closely do we in America approximate this ideal?

Proper education of every citizen in personal hygiene (*apart from the infectious diseases*) is scarcely even foreshadowed by existing efforts.

Medical supervision (*apart from the pauper, the criminal, and the insane*) is limited to a small portion only, of the school children only, in a few cities only; and does not pretend to remedy defects, but only to detect them.[5]

[5] About two-thirds of the children of America live and attend school in rural districts where medical supervision for defects is hardly yet more than contemplated.

Treatment of disease (*except for the pauper, the criminal, and the insane*) is a matter of private purchase or of private philanthropy, usually the private philanthropy of the private practicing physician.

The supervision of infectious persons is alone really established, authorized, or organized as a recognized duty of the State throughout America, and then only so far as the protection of others is concerned. We have not yet reached the treatment of the sick even though they be sick of infectious disease.

But the mechanism for even the function of preventing infection, although it is actually in existence, actually organized, actually authorized, actually operating, and has behind it long years of legal precedence and the support of public opinion, is sadly under-manned, and under-equipped,— merely a skeleton.

IMMEDIATE POSSIBILITIES

It is true that even those advanced States which have organized, in part or in whole, the above outlined operations, organized the control of infectious disease far earlier and more completely than they organized any of the others notwithstanding that that organization is usually inadequate in principle and inefficient in practice. They have done so in accordance with a general rule, which governs all mankind, namely, that of doing first the simplest, crudest, and most obviously necessary thing.

NON-INFECTIOUS DISEASES 43

But it is also a matter of fact that the supervision of infectious persons differs essentially in principles, methods, object, extent of application, and destiny, from education in personal hygiene, medical supervision for defects, or medical treatment. The latter are obviously, directly and immediately to and for the benefit of the individual who is educated, supervised, or treated. In principle, they are wise, fore-sighted and economic additions by the State to the welfare of its individual citizens. But the former is not to the benefit, usually rather to the temporary detriment, of the individual who comes under its operation. Its benefits are wholly to others, and even so do not add anything to their welfare, but merely prevent subtraction from it.

The methods of the infectious-disease supervisor are necessarily those of the detective and the policeman, not those of the educator or the medical supervisor. The object he seeks is prevention, not construction or even repair. He does not deal equally with every citizen for that citizen's good, as does the educator or the physician, but he ferrets out those few individuals who must be restrained for the good of the others. His destiny is, if successful, to eliminate the only reasons for his own official existence, while the educator and the medical supervisor will always continue to find in each new annual crop of children a new and constantly increasing field for their services.

In brief, the first three activities are, like boards of

public works, constructional in essence. Supervision of infection is, like the work of fire departments, conservative merely.

But although we may accept these four items as entirely proper for ultimate realization, we must acknowledge that the present public-health situation cannot be met merely by handing the outline over to boards of health or health departments as they exist to-day, notwithstanding that these departments constitute, by tradition and precedent, practice and organization, that arm of the government to which have been assigned the only activities of the State in relation to bodily welfare so far seriously or widely recognized.

Health departments in general are under-manned, under-equipped, continually distracted with futilities like garbage collection, the smoke nuisance, abolition of unnecessary noise and other simple police matters of an administrative character. But if expanded, their distractions eliminated, and their faces set sternly to the reduction of disease and death, they could not at once assume all the items of this program. Why?

The treatment of every citizen for all defects, disabilities and diseases we may dismiss from consideration at present. It is out of the question for some years to come in this country, despite the development reached in England.

For the education of every citizen in personal hygiene the basic necessities,— knowledge, authority, and organization,— are all lacking. For the supervision of

NON-INFECTIOUS DISEASES

every citizen for the detection (not the treatment) of defects, etc., knowledge, authority, and equipment can be had, it is true, although they may not be immediately available, but such detection of defects is closely bound up with treatment and should not be divorced from it, except as a method of demonstrating the need for treatment.

Only for the supervision of infectious diseases have we *now* all three,— knowledge, authority and equipment, although the latter merely in outline.

EDUCATION

Furthermore, it is true that the education of every citizen in personal hygiene, cannot be carried out properly (*apart from the prevention of certain diseases*) by *any* organization at the present time.

Why? Because such education requires, first, the knowledge, digestion, and formulation of the facts to be taught; and, second, the training of those who are to do the teaching.

But the best of us do not know personal hygiene (*apart from the prevention of certain diseases*); that is, we do not know how to care for and operate the human body as a machine. What, for instance, should be taught concerning diet when Chittenden and Wiley promulgate exactly opposite views? What should be taught concerning ventilation when the whole subject is but just emerging from chaos? What should be taught concerning clothing, sleep, exercise, and fatigue?

Our physiologists study the normal body, but more in relation to disease than to health. Our vital statisticians seek the factors of morbidity, not of physical perfection. Even the famous Federal "poison squad" sought to determine what is bad for people to eat, not what is good for them. All of these things are, of course, useful, excellent, even essential to know; but they do not teach us personal health, they teach only the avoidance of actual disease.

The truth is, that, as regards human bodily welfare, personal hygiene proper, we know, well enough to teach authoritatively, but one factor, that is the disease factor. We know disease because we have studied it. We know, it is true, the "personal hygiene" of farm animals because we have studied the "personal hygiene" of farm animals, at a cost of many million dollars a year. But we know nothing of the personal hygiene of human citizens, because we do not study the subject at all, except the hygiene of infants. We shall never know the personal hygiene of humans, apart, always, from the prevention of certain diseases, until we do study it — until we put as much time, pains, and money into it as any agricultural experimental station in any State puts into the study of the "personal hygiene" of farm animals. True it is a far more difficult subject, but that is the very reason why it requires immensely more study and experiment.

We recognize that the study of animal hygiene requires care, trained investigators, years of experiment.

NON-INFECTIOUS DISEASES 47

Why should we assume that the current dicta of those who pose as preachers of hygiene without study or special knowledge should be all sufficient in the case of the human?

There is, however, no real reason why health departments should teach personal hygiene at all, *apart from the prevention of disease,* any more than that they should teach personal morals or personal finance. Health departments have no peculiar knowledge of the one any more than of the others; and if they had, there are professional teachers much more competent and possessing far greater facilities than any health department.

Education concerning even infectious diseases is not strictly health-department work. This, like personal hygiene, should be taught seriously and systematically in the public schools. Ninety per cent. of the population never enter high schools, and only 1 per cent. reach the university. Whatever of personal hygiene or prevention of infection the citizen should know, must be taught in the grades or miss its mark. No amount of desultory pamphleteering or lecturing by health departments can ever take the place of properly conducted grade courses. Unlike courses in personal hygiene, about which we know next to nothing, courses in the prevention of infection could be established at once, since we know almost all about it; but it is no part of health-department work to conduct such courses. Health departments are police bodies, not preachers or teachers. They may well, it is true, educate the educators. There is no reason why they should educate the public, except the failure of the professional educators to do so.

MEDICAL SUPERVISION OF SCHOOLS

Medical supervision of school children, so far as it deals with defects, deals with non-transmissible conditions. Medical supervision, so far as it deals with infection, deals with transmissible conditions. The latter therefore detects links in the chain of the ramifying threads of infection throughout the community,— a ramification, the threads of which unquestionably should be in health-department hands.

But medical supervision for infectious disease in school as a means for general control of all infections has had a singularly exaggerated importance attached to it. Only one-half of the State's children attend school in any one year, and even the school child passes but one-ninth of each year in school. Were health departments alert in their familiarity with, and efficient in their control of, the ramifications of the chains of infection outside of the schools, they would locate and supervise the infective child before, not after, he had infected school children; before, not after, the medical supervisors for defects discovered him in the class-room. This would be accomplished incidentally to the control of infectious diseases amongst children below and above school age, as well as in adults.

NON-INFECTIOUS DISEASES

The fact is that medical supervision for defects *need* never encounter infection in that one-fourth of the total population which is contained in the schools, if health departments did their work properly in the other three-fourths which is outside of the schools. But this fact carries, alas, no guarantee that infective children will not, for a long time to come, occupy a share of the medical school supervisors' attention because, for a long time to come, health departments will not effectively control infection, inside or outside of schools, unless present methods are radically readjusted and expanded. Especially will this be true in rural districts where nearly two-thirds of the children secure their education and where health-department organization and equipment is, practically speaking, non-existent.

Hence, whatever may be our individual views with regard to the ultimate relation of medical school-supervision for defects to supervision of infectious persons, we need not blind ourselves to the fact that ideal conditions are far in the future, and that immediate necessities call for immediate adjustments which may be temporary or not, depending on future developments.

Medical supervision for defects and medical supervision for infection are now, and for some time to come must remain, so interdependent that the closest co-operation, even, in the rural districts, amalgamation, will be necessary. Such amalgamation should be under health departments, wherever that is possible, rather than under school boards.

First, because school boards have no authority through tradition, from precedence or by law, as have health departments to follow, outside of the schools, the ramifications of infection of which the infective child in the school constitutes but one link, nor even to follow that one link back to its home.

Second, because school boards have no information or authority concerning the full half of the children who are not of school age nor concerning any adult except those directly connected with the schools.

Finally, amalgamation in the rural districts is essential for one great reason, if for no other, and this reason is that if we do not combine both functions in one, in the rural districts, we shall not secure either function there at all.

SUMMARY

Non-infectious diseases, disabilities, and defects constitute a field for governmental attention as great as or greater than do the infectious diseases.

There are no theoretical reasons why governments should not concern themselves with the greater (the non-infectious group), as well as with the lesser (the infectious group).

Public-health activities in their very broadest conception would include all the functions of government, since there is nothing of interest to man, from high finance to municipal playgrounds, which has not some relation to health.

NON-INFECTIOUS DISEASES

But an administrative system so vast as to control all human activities related to health would merely replace the government, and would itself be necessarily subdivided, much as existing governments are now.

It is not difficult to outline a logical program for one branch of any government, a branch which should deal with the bodily welfare of man and include hygienic education, medical supervision, medical treatment, and the suppression of infectious diseases.

But there are many practical, as well as theoretical, reasons why health departments will not, indeed cannot, proceed at once to put this program into execution. Concerning education in personal hygiene, *apart from the infectious diseases,* agreement as to the basic facts to be taught has yet to be reached. As to the second and third items, organization, broad precedent, and broad authority are all lacking.

Concerning the infectious diseases, and concerning them only, are the paths clear and the duties plain.

The " instant need of things " is to do faithfully and well that one duty which we fully understand, the only one for which organization, authority, tradition, precedent, and the support of public opinion are already in our hands, i.e., the abolition of infectious diseases. To this end, the embryonic beginnings of the medical supervision of every citizen — that is, medical school-supervision — should lend its aid, especially in the rural districts.

But until we have accomplished this — the simplest,

easiest, crudest of our obvious and recognized duties, that one which lies right at our finger-tips — we cannot very well ask that the Nation should hand over to health departments all its great problems of life, death, health, and national development.

To achieve the abolition of infection we must strip for action, discard all useless armor and antiquated weapons, cease desultory bombardment at leisurely long range of the enemy's outlying domains, and personally seek, with well-shortened weapons, the enemy himself (infection) in his real stronghold (the infective person).

CHAPTER VI

EDUCATIONAL MECHANISM

The teaching of these new principles of Public Health must begin with the teaching of the teachers. Until our leading public health men, physicians, physiologists, and clergy acknowledge these teachings and give them their endorsement the old misleading statements, household traditions, worn-out dicta, now constituting the baseless platitudes of most public health beliefs, will remain false beacon lights leading nowhere.

It is time for all such leaders to awake and ask themselves whence these teachings came. They are not in our books; they are not propagated by our leading men of science. For instance no student of the subject has said a word to make any one believe that young children die of infections in less proportions than older children do, but quite the contrary. Yet in the face of all the books, all studies on the subject, all figures of statistics ever gathered, the medical profession itself in large proportions repeats the worn out sophistry: let them have it early and get it over — youth is the safest time; just as it repeats many another misconception not less malignant in its evil leading. That typhoid fever is a filth **disease** and due to general dirt, has been exploded for many years, yet we hear this statement made on every hand. Typhoid fever is not by any means carried by water only, yet this bit of knowledge seems still unknown to many leaders, even public health men. That the weak contract disease more than the strong one hears proclaimed from every pulpit, clerical or lay — but asked for their authority these proclaimers quote only the word of mouth of some physician who in turn can find only untraced tradition as his authority.

Once leaders are agreed, the next most necessary step will be a revision of the teachings in Normal Schools; and this necessitates the preparation of books on hygiene that will place in proper perspective all the real health measures that we have and show just what each one will do. The public must be trusted with the facts. The timid soul holds back the truth that bathing does not prevent disease, that lack of bathing does not end in sudden death, because forsooth he fears the children may come dirty to his school! He forgets that the children often come dirty now, in spite of all his teaching; true many others are clean, but both escape disease or suffer from it quite irrespective of the number of their baths. They who bathe from fear of death are few, and we must reach clean bodies by some other route than bogies held up with orotund words, bogies whose pumpkin heads and candle-sputtered light the listeners sense although they may not see the mechanism. Honesty in teaching is as necessary in our public health as in our mathematics or geography.

Let us face frankly this; about the body-care we know few facts of practical application to our everyday life that are really hygienic, not merely æsthetic. We know of course we should not be, for high efficiency, too hot, too cold, too wet, too dry, too hungry or too full. We should not sleep too long, nor sleep too little, work too hard, or loaf, and so on; but to say what is too much or too little for any given person, especially to lay down the golden mean, is something no one knows. The individual variations in individuals are very great; what is too hard work for one will scarcely stir the blood of another. " What is meat for one is another's poison." These variations are partly inherent; the exposure to cold which would be disastrous for the negro or even the white man is likely to suit the Inuit exactly; but also previous training and experience affect exercise and sleep and diet, etc., by the establishment of compensations, for the range of adaptation of the body to variations is very great: finally it seems probable that the following out of any exact " ideal " regimen would be in itself far from ideal, for it would do away with those very variations which, by cultivating compensations, maintain the body in its best state of general efficiency to meet the inevitable physiological emergencies of daily life.

That such an ideal regimen would be far from ideal because of its utter impracticability for the great mass of the race seems seldom to occur to those who advocate the search for it. The great mass of the work-a-day world must now and for long generations yet to come eat, sleep, work, etc., not as they would but as they can.

It is of course true that the excesses and the deprivations from which so many people suffer are so extreme as to be obviously harmful often even to themselves and quite obviously so to those acquainted with any sort of good bodily condition. But these extremes are often either results of poverty or, curiously enough, results of choice upon the part of those concerned, particularly in sleep, diet, and work. The race as a whole does not desire efficiency in practice, but chiefly excitement or amusement. To these ends, substituted in many minds for the more worthy pursuit of happiness, much of the lack of hygiene exemplified by the excesses and the deprivations may be traced, rather than to real necessity.

The great preacher urging on his flock the highest ideals, often breaks down himself from over-strain, thus failing to practice what he preaches every day. The physician, the lawyer, the teacher, often neglectfully or deliberately break the simplest rules prescribing the most liberal limits for bodily success.

Hence the educational campaign for hygiene, i.e., for bodily efficiency, must be antedated by or combined with a general reconstruction of ideals not based on mere intensity, but on all-round development; and these must be so shaped that every one may have within his ready grasp the opportunities for such a life that the extremes are not forced on him by circumstances taking their roots in the foundations of society itself.

Hygiene then in its practical application to the world at large is something still far in the future, requiring as a rule the reconstruction of individual but far more of communal life. As yet we do not so study the body of the human in our physiology as to determine what are the ideal conditions. We are beginning to do so; and for our public institutions some sort of rules of thumb relating to clothing, exercise, and diet are traced out to meet the average wants. But who that knows our institutions would dare claim that the conduct of them really meets the bodily demands of all their inmates or brings them to the highest point of physical efficiency? Too often, outside of armies, this is not by any means the ideal held in mind. In most institutions keeping down expense is the chief object; in our industrial operations the commercial output is the goal, not the condition of the factory hands. True it is that public health, in the division which deals with hygiene (efficiency with comfort, and long life for all), must rest upon the attainment of the ideals sought by many sociological movements for the mental and moral recasting of the race. No movement which has for an object the proper understanding of man or of any of his relations to the world can fail to be helpful in some way to this end.

But when we turn to the second great item of public health, the prevention of disease, we find a different situation. True, as has been already explained, proper hygiene necessarily eliminates certain diseases which arise from improper living, accidents, the effects of monotonous repetitions of the same movements, or the monotonous maintenance of the same positions; certain non-living poisons; and the internal disruptions and disabilities due to excesses and deprivations. The education needed to eliminate these must in itself be specific; although the realization of their abolition must be the result of improvements in general social and trade conditions. Accidents occur amongst millionaires as well as amongst factory hands; lead poisoning, phosphorous poisoning, alcoholism, etc., depend after all upon taking those poisons into the body. They cannot occur under the worst sociological conditions, not even in the utter barbarism of the Central African village, unless those poisons enter into the system. The most important of all the preventable diseases, the infectious, are likewise due to specific poisons; but poisons alive, living and breeding in human bodies. No sociological advances, no moral developments, no improvement in living or in the relations of man to man, no raising of the standards of surroundings, no highest care of the body or attention to its efficiency can evade these unless the specific germ is evaded; which means evading the contact of uninfected man with infected man. But all sociological, moral and mental advance tend to cultivate contact, to bring all classes of people closer together, to knit the social fabric into more interdependent and mutually helpful structures.

Industrial advances gathering together larger and larger groups of people engaged in the same enterprises result in more and more social intercourse in masses, especially well knit if moral and mental development of the groups is sought. The public schools tend to more and more getting together, to wider interests, to the closer affiliation of each individual with every other. Improved transportation, the essential to national growth, has as its avowed object the extension of contact of one with another. The specific poisons of the specific infectious diseases are transmitted by this contact. So long as such contact continues, much more as it is extended, these diseases will be more and more widely spread, unless the specific poisons themselves, which are bred in human bodies and transferred in human discharges, can be themselves eliminated. The hope that the remodeling of human conduct, the education of the race to protect each other by the elimination of the exchange of these discharges, is negatived by the character of the exchange. True in the illicit venereal diseases the form of contact most often operative to propagate these diseases is a form of contact which is not essential to ordinary business or social relations and can be voluntarily ended. But the moral and mental development of the race as a whole to the point where this form of contact is eliminated cannot be hoped for in many years to come. Like alcoholism, venereal diseases will be contracted so long as the specific cause is to be had. In the "children's diseases," each new crop of children, each theoretically amenable to training in self protection, contract these diseases before they can be trained. Finally the technique of self protection and of protection of others through the skillful limitation of the spread of discharges is a technique acquirable only after months of rigid training by those devoted to the especial studies and work connected with it, in contagious hospitals, so that even highly trained experts dealing with infections contract them at times; and when themselves infected find it immensely difficult to protect others unless they too are trained. Education directed to the vanquishment of these diseases must therefore be education pointing out the specific sources, the impossibility of the protection against them by any form of conduct practicable in ordinary life, and the necessity for the elimination of the infection itself. This elimination means the search for and the restriction of the small number of infected persons existing at any given time, with the object of eliminating infection from them and restoring them to the communal life when free of danger to the community. The mechanisms needed to discover these infected persons, a general agreement that their temporary segregation is essential, a mutual helpfulness in discovering them and in assisting those charged with that duty, all these can be secured by education. But the actual doing of the work itself must rest in the hands of experts armed with full authority, pursuing their ends with quiet persistence and largely without spectacular show or noise.

EDUCATIONAL MECHANISM 61

To the extent to which the discovery and temporary segregation of the infected may remove these infected individuals from the communal life, such operations will benefit the communal life; and the provision for the care and maintenance of those thus segregated and of those dependant on them must be a communal charge. But the community would gain so immensely in efficiency and comfort and long life by the segregation of the infected, because of the thus obtained elimination of disease and death from the uninfected that the expense of suffering, disease, and death, existing now, might well be thus diverted to the purpose of escaping both.

SUMMARY

The education of the public in personal hygiene, the development and efficiency of the body, must, like all other effective education, be carried out through the public schools; although immense service may be done by educational propaganda in the magazines and newspapers, which now form the postgraduate schools of the race.

The elimination of those diseases which depend upon the physical surroundings must be a matter of specific training of those who come in contact with those specific surroundings in such sociological improvements as may eliminate their existence. In the infectious diseases the poisons are not definite visible labeled things but, to the ordinary citizen, invisible and undetectable.

They are not limited to certain kinds or forms of surroundings but exist in human beings themselves. They can be found only by specific methods and the conditions under which they are transmitted cannot be so sufficiently altered in practical everyday life as to restrict their transmission by private effort. The infectious diseases therefore are peculiarly matters for direct Governmental control; and the Governmental measures undertaken must be planned and carried out, not merely to hold them in abeyance, but to secure their absolute abolition.

CHAPTER VII

THE OLD PRACTICE AND THE NEW

EPIDEMIOLOGY

THE previous chapters were designed to clear the way for the constructive program which the following chapters seek to set forth.

The conclusion so far reached is that the chief immediate duty of official public health is the abolition of all the infectious diseases. For this great enterprise, both scientific principles and scientific practice are essential. The new public health principles have been outlined; the new public health practice remains to be explained.

Public health practice in handling infectious diseases may be traced through three distinct eras: past, present, and future.

Past, or era of " general sanitation."— The practice followed energetically in epidemics, spasmodically and perfunctorily at other times, consisted in a strenuous campaign of " general cleaning up "; an orgy of sweeping, burning, scrubbing; an ecstasy of dirt-destruction, individual, household, municipal.[1]

[1] The reader is begged, pleaded with, besought, not to repeat at this point the wearisome old gibe — Then you want us to live

This "general sanitation" was a true old-style shotgun prescription, used discriminately for any outbreak of any disease. No distinction of *sources* from *routes* of infection was made; indeed, that a distinction existed was hardly recognized, and, looking back, it sometimes seems that even the most obvious relations of cause and effect often were ignored.

Present, or era of " specific sanitation."— The best practice now is deliberately to analyze the particular outbreak of the particular disease concerned; speedily to determine thus the exact *route* of infection actually responsible; and promptly to abolish or block that route.

Future, or era of " supervision of sources."— The practice, so far as it is possible to forecast it, will be the location and supervision of the *sources* of infection (infected persons) before, not after, they gain access to *routes;* thus in time eliminating infectious diseases entirely.

like pigs? If not, why do you condemn "general sanitation"? We do not condemn "general sanitation," or cleanliness, or order, or decency. We simply present the scientific fact that these things do not greatly prevent, nor does their absence produce, infectious diseases. They have a thousand advantages, but not this one. Honesty does not protect against lightning; yet this fact cannot prevent any truly honest man from remaining honest, nor does its statement in the least detract from the true virtues of honesty. And so with "general sanitation." It is *specific*, not "general," cleanliness that prevents infection. Specific cleanliness is that directed, not broadly and blindfold against all "dirt," but scientifically and efficiently against the one "dirt" (infected matter) that produces disease.

THE OLD PRACTICE AND THE NEW 65

It will be noted that public health practice as thus outlined, past, present, and future, forms a definitely developing mechanism, concentrating itself by degrees from the general to the particular, from the surroundings to the individual, from (a) the random application of blanket measures, through (b) a specific detection and a specific correction of a specific bad condition, to (c) the actual forestalling of the development of such conditions at all.

COMPARATIVE METHODS

To make clear this most important matter of public health practice, illustrations follow, exhibiting the public health practice of the different eras as each would operate in the face of a typhoid fever epidemic; typhoid being selected because the control of this one disease alone calls for almost every modern public health principle, and, in some form, every modern public health practice.

The end sought was, is, and always will be, the same, — to stop the spread of the disease.

But the methods of the different eras contrast widely.

In the past era of "general sanitation," a typhoid epidemic was met by a vigorous attack on dirt, damp cellars, dust, disorder; on garbage, manure, dead animals, weeds, defective plumbing, and stagnant pools; cobwebs were cleared away; windows were opened to "let in the blessed sunshine"; preachers preached cleanliness; teachers taught bathing; health officers limed back alleys and whitewashed outhouses. Human nature demanded "action," and "action," of a kind, was supplied. As a rule, the outbreak ran for weeks or months despite all that was done, exhausted the material available to feed it, and died out as any fire will if all the fuel is burned up. Whichever of the "methods" for control happened to be instituted last received the credit of conquering the outbreak, although none of them had, as a rule, the slightest effect.

We know now, what our forefathers did not know then, that typhoid infection is carried by water, food, flies, milk, and contact, and that "general cleaning up" could not remove infection from polluted water-mains, or purify a contaminated milk supply; could not stop the eating of infected food or eliminate contact infection.[2] The only form of typhoid outbreak which "general sanitation" could at all affect was the form due to flies[3] carrying infected matter from accumulations

[2] Contact infection is the infection which radiates directly from the infected person through nose and mouth and bladder and bowel discharges. The hands of the infector and of his associates are the chief carriers of all these discharges, although mouth-spray and sputum also act in many diseases. Things directly infected by these discharges are also dangerous, but practically only while the discharges remain fresh and moist. The radius of action of contact is usually small; it compares with the radius of action of water, food, flies, and milk somewhat as a bayonet compares with a machine gun in a general mêlée. But contact infection in the long run is more deadly than other routes, for there are many "bayonets" to each one such "machine gun."

[3] We do not now use "general sanitation" even for fly out-

THE OLD PRACTICE AND THE NEW

of exposed bowel discharges, usually from non-fly proof toilets. In so far as the efforts at general sanitation may have had, at times, some remote and indirect effect on reducing the number of flies or separating them from the infected discharges, "general sanitation" may have at times had some partial and inadequate but still more or less helpful results. But of course the fly was not then known as a route of infection in typhoid, so that even the results that "general sanitation" secured were secured largely by accident, i.e., by the unrecognized conjunction of an unappreciated remedy with an undetermined cause.

The present era of "specific sanitation" began a decade or so ago. Water, food, flies, and milk have gradually become fully recognized as the main public routes of typhoid infection, i.e., as the main routes from individual to group, and from group to group; contact, especially of late, has been recognized as the great private route, i.e., from individual to individual. Outbreaks have been met chiefly by finding the particular route involved, and by abolishing or blocking that route. But even in this era, the earlier practice for the attainment of this end differed fundamentally from that of to-day.

breaks. From this old shot-gun prescription we have eliminated all the ingredients but one, that one which alone was active. In fly outbreaks we exclude flies from infected discharges, and (so far as the primary outbreak is concerned) then stop. So does the outbreak.

The earlier epidemiologists [4] of this era argued thus: "Water, food, flies, and milk are the known public routes; usually some one of these routes is responsible in each outbreak. Therefore, to find the responsible route in any given instance, flood the stricken community with trained inspectors; analyze the water supplies; investigate the milk supplies; go through the markets; delve into the provision stores; estimate the number of flies, and locate their breeding-places; survey the back alleys and out-door toilets; plat all results on maps; interview the city engineer, the fire marshal, the meat and milk inspectors, and examine their official records; secure the morbidity and mortality records of the board of health; study all available meteorological, topographical, geological, and other data; in brief, probe, dissect, tabulate, collate, and compare all possible *physical* information concerning the community. Under such inquisition the guilty route of infection can scarcely escape detection."

For these methods it must be said that they were scientific, logical, and exhaustive; but they were terribly laborious and generally exceedingly slow. Of course it sometimes happened that the guilty route of infection was stumbled on at once; and almost always this end was reached sooner or later, too often, however, only after weeks, months, or even years of effort. The ponderous slowness of these methods took them out of the class of effective emergency measures, and

[4] Experts on epidemics.

THE OLD PRACTICE AND THE NEW

this was recognized even then, for a typhoid investigation was not then considered a matter of haste, in initiation or in execution.

These earlier methods parallel somewhat those which we might suppose an amateur hunter to use, if he were commissioned to find a certain sheep-killing wolf. Confronted with this problem, the amateur might, not unreasonably, flood the surrounding mountains with assistants, instructing them to find all the existing wolf-trails, and to follow each such trail inward towards the slaughtered sheep until satisfied that it did, or did not, actually lead to them.

The methods of to-day are the exact converse of these. Instead of finding in the mountains and following inward from them, say, 500 different wolf trails, 499 of which must necessarily be wrong, the experienced hunter goes directly to the slaughtered sheep, finding there and following outward thence the only right trail,— the only trail that is there,— the one trail that is necessarily and inevitably the trail of the one actually guilty wolf.

THE NEW EMERGENCY EPIDEMIOLOGY

The epidemiologist of to-day, called to a typhoid-stricken community, at first pays no attention at all to the *physical* condition of the existing possible routes. It is sociological data, not physical, that he needs at this stage. He knows that, counting the wells, the toilets, the milk supplies, etc., there may be 500 of these possible routes; but he does not go to see them, nor even the pumping-station or the sewage-outfall. He goes, hot foot, straight to the "slaughtered sheep" — straight to the patient's bedside. There, and there only, can he expect to find the trail of the guilty wolf — the route by which the infection reached that patient. There, in thirty minutes, he reduces the 500 *possibilities* to, say, 10, i.e., to those encountered (a) *by this patient*[5] (b) *at a certain time* (the date of his infection). These 10 are carefully listed; but the epidemiologist does not investigate even these 10. He goes, instead, straight to another bedside and lists there the, say, 10 routes that constitute the possible routes for this second patient; but he does not investigate the routes on this list either; *he merely compares the two lists.* Why? Because the one guilty route quite evidently must be on *both* lists. Thus if both lists show the same water supply, that water supply remains a possible guilty route; but, if not, *water is eliminated.* If both lists show the same milk supply, that milk supply remains a possible guilty route; but, if not, *milk is eliminated.* Discarding thus the routes not common to both lists, 5 routes, say, still remain. At the third patient's bedside these 5 are reduced by similar treatment, to say, 3. So the search goes on until the epidemiologist either locates the one main public route

[5] Of course imported and secondary cases are not used for this purpose, and at this stage the epidemiologist is most careful to eliminate all such from his tabulations.

THE OLD PRACTICE AND THE NEW 71

common to all or proves that the outbreak is not due to such a public route at all, but to the private routes extending directly from person to person, i.e., to contact. Often in twelve hours of such work, generally in twenty-four, almost always in thirty-six, the evidence is conclusive. The guilty route stands out convicted; for it is found on every list, and the innocent routes are exonerated, for they occur only on some.[6]

STOPPING A "PRIMARY" EPIDEMIC

Now, at last, and not till now, does the epidemiologist deal directly with the route of infection thus indicated, examine it to find just how it is responsible, including the source of its infection, and thus provide the initial data for its remedy.[7] These remedies consist broadly

[6] Obviously this method fails if there be but one patient, for then comparison of lists is of course impossible; but single cases usually prove to be imported or from contact. Also it may happen that even three or four patients do not furnish sufficient data to narrow the possible routes to one; obviously, the more patients there are the more conclusive the results. But even when only a few patients exist, this method reduces the number of routes to be investigated to say, 10, often to 2 or 3, an immense reduction from the original 500.

[7] To those who are not familiar with modern public health work, this account may seem incredible or at least exaggerated, yet these are the regular procedures of emergency epidemiology wherever they are understood to-day. Records of such work in America for years back are open to all enquirers. Moreover, the above account has pictured the epidemiologist working under a most disadvantageous condition, i.e., in complete ignorance of the community he deals with, except for what he learns during the investigation itself. If previous familiarity

in one of two general procedures — the prevention of further infection of the guilty route — or, if this cannot be accomplished, the installation of some method of removing the infection after it has been unavoidably admitted. The former method is "the abolition of the source," the latter "the blocking of the route." As illustrations of the former may be cited the diversion of an infected feeder from an otherwise pure water supply; the disinfection of the discharges of typhoid patients before deposit in outdoor toilets; the elimination from a milk-business of a typhoid-carrying employee; in brief, the prevention of infection of the public routes by elimination of the sources of infection, which are typhoid-infected discharges. As examples of the blocking of routes may be cited the boiling, the chemical disinfection, or the filtration of a polluted water supply; the pasteurization of infected milk; the disinfection of the hands of those who are typhoid-carriers or who handle the typhoid-infected discharges of others.

The simplicity, effectiveness, and inexpensiveness of the abolition of sources as compared with the blocking of routes is evident on a moment's consideration. Yet with the affected community exists, the main public route of infection can often be determined without leaving headquarters, provided merely that correct data as to the number, location, and dates of infection of the cases are submitted. Of course such "long-distance epidemiology," wonderfully accurate though it can be made, does not compare in reliability or in finish of detail with actual personal investigation on the ground.

THE OLD PRACTICE AND THE NEW 73

in the slow development of human knowledge and appreciation of their relative values, the latter are still relied upon as a rule almost to the exclusion of the former.

It is at the point when the guilty public route is shown (if public route there be) that the epidemiologist, so far as this public route is concerned, steps out, and the bacteriologist, the chemist, the sanitary engineer step in; one, or any two, or all three, as conditions may require. It is they who at the present time and as a rule must work out the most available methods of (a) immediately ending present danger; (b) permanently providing against its recurrence.

STOPPING "SECONDARY" OUTBREAKS

But detecting and demonstrating the guilt of a main public route, when such is involved, by no means ends the epidemiologist's duties. The work outlined so far is required (in America) chiefly in typhoid outbreaks; and then chiefly in those typhoid outbreaks which are derived from water, food, flies, or milk. The work still to be done is required in *all* typhoid outbreaks, whether initially derived from these public routes or from contact; moreover, it is called for in the majority of outbreaks of all the *other* infectious diseases, because the majority are usually contact outbreaks at *all* stages. That work is *the prevention of further spread by contact*.

To understand this clearly, it must be remembered

that under present conditions every typhoid, or other, epidemic which *begins* from some one public route (water, food, flies, or milk) soon presents two distinct parts; the primary outbreak, consisting of that group of persons who received their infection wholesale through the public route; and the secondary outbreak, consisting of those individuals who later, by the private routes of contact, receive their infection individually and directly from the individuals of the primary set. Those typhoid, or other, epidemics which *begin* through the private routes of contact, i.e., when one infected individual succeeds in directly infecting a large group, do not, of course, present a " primary " outbreak at all. They are, so to put it, " secondary " outbreaks from the outset. (Of course, it will be understood that these distinctions are somewhat artificial and for convenience. The so-called primary outbreak affecting wholesale a group of persons through a public route of infection such as a public water supply, milk, etc., does not truly originate with the water, milk, etc., which is involved. A previous case or group of cases must of course have infected the water or milk. Typhoid fever is not generated by these or any other *routes;* they act merely as transmitters from person or persons to person or persons. The chain of infection therefore reaches back into the past indefinitely to the hypothetical day, indefinite ages gone, when the typhoid germ first appeared upon the stage of the world's history.)

The search for a public route is therefore only the

THE OLD PRACTICE AND THE NEW 75

first step in subduing any epidemic. If such route exist, this step, by finding it, provides for getting rid of it, which prevents the infection of any more persons from that route, and so ends the primary outbreak. But this first step by no means ends the epidemic as a whole, for the persons already infected from that public route constitute each one a source of further spread by contact, a spread which, of course, must also be prevented. Obviously, epidemics which are contact epidemics throughout, necessarily present an identical problem from this standpoint, for every existing infected person, whatever the route of his infection, is a separate danger, and each requires supervision.[8]

FINDING THE UNKNOWN CASES

How does the prevention of further spread by contact infection from existing cases depend on epidemiology? Cannot the spread of infection by contact from existing

[8] In earlier days the fallacy that typhoid fever patients could not directly infect their associates — in brief, that typhoid fever was not contagious — was responsible for the long-delayed recognition of secondary typhoid outbreaks, even after the origin of primary outbreaks had been learned and methods of dealing with them perfected. We know now that abolishing or blocking a primary route is but half the story. The primary cases, if neglected, may continue to infect other persons by contact, and these again others, ad infinitum. Such secondary outbreaks may extend slowly for months or years and yield cases equaling or exceeding in number those from the primary outbreak. The "endemic typhoid" of some localities is at times an unrecognized, slow-moving, secondary outbreak.

cases be guarded against by the attendants (nurses and physicians) which each such case (*if known*) necessarily has? True, and were these *known* cases the only danger-points, proper attention to preventing spread from them would be all-sufficient. But the *known* cases usually form but half of the danger-points because only half of the dangerously infected persons become *known* cases. The other half consists of "missed cases" (mild, unrecognized, and concealed cases, early cases, and, later on, convalescing cases) and of "carriers." (The "carriers" are infected persons, capable of infecting others, but not themselves made ill by the disease germs which they nevertheless carry and distribute.)

Missed cases and carriers, *unless especially sought for,* are, and must necessarily remain, unknown to those capable of guarding them; they have no known attendants to whom the prevention of spread of infection from them can be entrusted; they generally do not know themselves to be infected; and, if ignored, they are more dangerous, because inevitably unguarded, than the known cases, for, being known, the latter can be guarded.

This problem, the finding of missed cases and carriers, is now solved by an epidemiological procedure which, while less spectacular, is far more widely useful than that of finding public routes, because it applies, not alone to contact-typhoid outbreaks, but to all contact outbreaks, that is, to all infectious diseases, from

THE OLD PRACTICE AND THE NEW 77

tuberculosis down. Were the ability to find *public routes* of infection in water, food, fly, and milk outbreaks the only virtue of epidemiology, its services, immense though they have been to the control of primary typhoid, could have no value in the great mass of infectious disease, for the great mass arises chiefly by contact. It is the ability to find the *private sources* of infection in *contact* outbreaks that makes epidemiology the pivotal factor of modern public health.

This location of missed cases and carriers in typhoid, and other, outbreaks, is called concurrent epidemiology, and is well worth thoroughly understanding. Its explanation will be found in the next chapter.

SUMMARY

Modern public-health practice for the control of infectious diseases consists, not in the *physical surveillance* of whole communities, but in the *sociological study* of the *infected persons* in them.

This practice is best illustrated in the modern handling of typhoid fever epidemics, because this disease is all-inclusive, i.e., it travels by all four of the great public routes (water, food, flies, and milk), as well as by the private fifth route, contact; also because typhoid is an intestinal infection and, of all the infectious diseases of the temperate zone, the intestinal infections *alone* travel by *all* of these five great routes.

A typhoid epidemic is approached, as is any other epidemic, first, to determine if any public route of infection is involved, and, if so, what that route is and how it operates, including often how it became infected in the first place; thus finding how to stop further infection of groups of people through it; second, to determine the private routes and *sources* of the contact outbreak from individual to individual which, sooner or later, develops in all epidemics, whether the original route be a public route or not.

To the epidemiologist, the public-health detective, falls all these crucial tasks. It is his function to find those underlying facts concerning the sources and routes of infection which alone can form a sound basis for real remedial measures.

How he performs the finding of *public routes* and often, of the sources of their infection, has been described; the finding of *private routes* and *sources* will be described later. In both procedures the initial step is the same, namely, the investigation of the known cases. By seeing and questioning *known* cases, or their immediate relatives and attendants, the epidemiologist can classify them into native and imported. The native cases, since they alone originated in the community under investigation, are further classified into primary and secondary cases. From the histories of the primary cases, if such there be, he learns the public route and provides thus the data for its abrogation. From *all* the cases, imported, primary, and secondary, he obtains the data needed for the next step.

CHAPTER VIII

THE NEWEST PRACTICE

CONCURRENT EPIDEMIOLOGY [1]

The preceding chapter outlined the first step in the modern handling of a typhoid fever epidemic, typhoid fever being selected because its proper handling illustrates best the principles and practice of modern public health work.

The first step is the discovery, by the methods of *emergency* epidemiology, whether water, food, flies, milk, or contact

[1] *Emergency* epidemiology is the epidemiology required in outbreaks from single great routes — water, food, flies, milk. *Concurrent* epidemiology is the epidemiology required in contact outbreaks, i.e., outbreaks from multiple private sources. Emergency epidemiology is rapid and spectacular; it is played hard, against time, to save large groups of people. Concurrent epidemiology is relatively slow and plodding; it ferrets out, one by one, the individual persons whose infection threatens families or small groups. Emergency epidemiology will disappear when the great routes are properly protected by purification methods or, even better, by such supervision of all cases that infection of such routes becomes impossible. Concurrent epidemiology will greatly develop; it is the most powerful and practical weapon yet devised for *the abolition of the infectious diseases* and hence for doing away with the necessity of guarding routes at all. To revert to the wolf parable, guarding the routes by which the wolves may reach the sheep is good, provided eternal vigilance and a uniformly high standard of efficiency are maintained. Abolition of the wolves themselves is far more conclusive, and would make unnecessary the burden of guarding the routes for all time.

be the original main route of infection. The second step, to be outlined in these pages, is the location, by the methods of *concurrent* epidemiology, of all the infected persons (known cases, missed cases, and carriers). These are located because each, regardless of the original route by which he himself became infected, forms a new center of infection for spread by contact which will continue the outbreak indefinitely until such transfer is stopped, accidentally, or by exhaustion of susceptible material.

It was further pointed out that neither emergency epidemiology nor concurrent epidemiology were limited in their application to typhoid fever; and that the ability of concurrent epidemiology to handle properly contact typhoid outbreaks, whether contact be the secondary or primary route, is a conclusive demonstration of its ability to handle all other infectious diseases, since these others, while spread by public routes to some extent, are, in the mass, contact infections chiefly. No dependence on the argument by analogy from typhoid fever to other diseases is needed, however; for these other diseases are now and have been for years past handled successfully by these very methods.

Most persons contemplating the problem of finding missed cases and carriers for the first time, pronounce it impossible; then suggest, as the only solution, a house-to-house canvass of the whole community, hastily adding that of course such a measure is quite impractical. As a matter of fact, the public health detective does at times use, and use successfully, exactly that " impractical " measure,— the house-to-house canvass. This house-to-house method is used in primary outbreaks from public routes, to locate *unreported* primary " known cases," and also to locate primary missed cases and carriers. It is necessary in such primary outbreaks because the distribution of *primary* missed cases and carriers, as well as of "known cases," is co-extensive with that of the guilty route. There is no other guide to their location, and therefore the whole distribution of the guilty route must be searched. But the need of such a canvass of *a whole community* seldom arises except in typhoid or other infectious intestinal outbreaks; and then only when the infection is spread by a route *common* to the whole community; and therefore practically only when the guilty route is a public water supply. In milk outbreaks, those who did not use the guilty milk need not be examined; and a similar statement is true also regarding food outbreaks. Fly outbreaks rarely affect a whole community unless the community be very small; and in small communities of course a general canvass is not difficult.

In the majority of epidemics, and because the majority of epidemics are due, not to great public routes, but to private contact, the finding of missed cases and carriers does not require even a partial house-to-house canvass. This is true of secondary typhoid, and other *secondary* outbreaks (which are contact outbreaks) as well as of the great majority of all outbreaks (since the majority are contact outbreaks only).

The reason why missed cases and carriers can be found in contact outbreaks without a house-to-house canvass depends upon a fact of which the true significance is not fully appreciated outside of epidemiological circles. It is this: such missed cases and carriers are not distributed at pure, blind random anywhere and everywhere throughout the community. *They occur in certain groups — and these groups can be located because they betray themselves through their connection with known cases. Hence the location of known cases locates these groups also.*[2]

This most important epidemiological principle is called the principle of *zones of infection*. It is the cardinal principle of *concurrent* epidemiology.

The principle of *zones of infection* was first clearly recognized in diphtheria epidemics, and its development and demonstration as a practical working rule depends, primarily, on diphtheria investigations;[3] but both principle and practice have now been established for all the well-studied epidemic diseases.

The epidemiologist,[4] in putting this principle into practice, locates first the known cases, and then searches

[2] It must not be supposed that these groups are confined to families, immediate neighbors, etc. Their true basis is sociological relationship, not mere physical propinquity. In a single scarlet fever outbreak originating in one community Dr. A. J. Chesley found the related sociological groups distributed in 3 States, involving 3 cities, 2 villages, and 24 townships in 10 counties. The Mankato typhoid fever outbreak of 1908 affected over 40 points outside of Mankato.

[3] Developed largely by Drs. F. F. Wesbrook, L. B. Wilson, and O. McDaniel in Minnesota.

[4] It must be evident that those private practising physicians who are not health officers, cannot, for many reasons well understood by the profession, do epidemiological work, emergency or concurrent, except in overwhelming outbreaks, where ordinary

THE NEWEST PRACTICE 83

the zones of infection, which they indicate, for missed cases and carriers. The methods of this search vary with each disease and are described in some detail in other chapters. Detective methods are used, illuminated by expert technical knowledge of each disease, its natural history, and the means, laboratory and clinical, of recognizing it, at every stage and under all disguises. Suffice it to say now that the finding of missed cases and carriers, as well as of known cases,— that is, of the very framework of the ramifying threads of the infectious disease,— is a problem not only solvable, but already solved, and already reduced to a routine basis. As an art, this concurrent epidemiology is somewhat more arduous and time-consuming than the art of emergency epidemiology, but it is thoroughly

conventions and social relations are temporarily foregone. Even those private practicing physicians who are also health officers, encounter difficulties and obstructions, ethical, social and conventional, which professional epidemiologists, who are not in private practice, do not meet. Hence in all outbreaks the physician finds that his most valuable functions consist in treating the sick and in advising protective measures to those who apply to him. Physicians also often combine, very successfully, to publish material or give public lectures of instructions during epidemics. But, after all, the chief service which the physician can render to official public health is the reporting of *known cases*. Known cases, as has been shown, are the basic datum-points for emergency epidemiology, i.e., for the finding of the routes of infection; and they are even still more important to concurrent epidemiology, i.e., in the study of the zones of infection. Epidemiology is greatly aided when the physician performs thoroughly this, his primary, public health duty.

practical and has been successfully followed for years past all over Minnesota, in an average of four to six epidemics every week.[5] The visiting nurse in "concurrent epidemiology," can be made a most valuable and efficient aid, to say nothing at present of the other and even more indispensable services in other directions which are within her especial province.

This principle of zones of infection applies to tuberculosis just as to any other infection spread by contact; indeed, the location of missed cases in tuberculosis (carriers in tuberculosis are hypothetical to date) offers less difficulty to modern epidemiology than the same problem in other infectious diseases.

FUTURE APPLICATIONS

So much for past and present practice.

Turning now to the future era of "supervision of sources," the principles and practice already described pave the way for appreciation of the probable developments. In reconsidering the wolf metaphor already outlined, every one will ask, and wisely, Why wait until some sheep are killed before we protect the others? Why not patrol the known routes by which the wolves reach the sheep; or, better, build wolf-proof folds; or, best of all, teach the sheep to protect themselves — to fight the wolves or at least to dodge them?

Those who believe that infectious disease can be

[5] See reports of the Minnesota State Board of Health for 1911 and 1913.

THE NEWEST PRACTICE 85

warded off, in the face of infection, by diet,[6] exercise, good ventilation, and " strict observance of the laws of bodily health," are those who would train the sheep to fight; would train the body to destroy all infection that

[6] A most important exception to the general statement that proper diet in itself cannot prevent the development of infection provided infection gains access to the body should be recorded to cover the case of nursing infants. It has long been noted that breast-fed infants, during the period that they are so fed (but during that period only) are, practically speaking, immune to many infectious diseases. This is so true of scarlet fever and measles, that in such diseases no great concern need be felt for such an infant, even though the mother herself have the disease. In diphtheria, a nursling to some extent shows a like immunity. In smallpox, this is not true and in tuberculosis it is at most very doubtful.

That this escape of nurslings is purely a matter of the enormous advantages in nutritional value, to an infant, of mother's milk over other foods has yet to be demonstrated. Nursing infants are by the mere fact of nursing less likely than are other infants to be exposed to whatever routes or sources of infection may be about, unless the mother is herself a source. But in scarlet fever and measles, at least, this is not the whole explanation. It has been suggested that the real reason lies in the transmission to the child of actual immunity-producing bodies in mother's milk. If this be so, breast-feeding in infants as a protection against certain infectious diseases combines in one operation three principles of defense; good nutrition, specific immunization and the avoidance of infection. Other forms of feeding fail to provide these defences; and usually combine against the infant poor nutrition, absence of immunization, and exposure to the five routes of infection. Great skill and care and constant watchfulness may serve in artificial feeding partially to offset these dangers; breast-feeding automatically protects against them almost without effort. Moreover, breast-feeding accomplishes in *other ways* four times the service in saving

may reach it. But, as we do not know how to teach sheep to fight, so we do not know the laws of health needed for this purpose if any such exist.[7] Such methods tested against infection have generally failed[8] so far. In that day when sheep fight wolves they may succeed.

Those who believe that the sheep may be taught to dodge the wolves have much more in their favor.

Dodging infection is well understood. The physician, the nurse, the epidemiologist, handle with impunity the very sources of infection themselves,— infected persons and their infected discharges. Why not teach this art to every citizen? The principle is simple,— prevent infected discharges from entering the mouth. It is in the practising of this principle, simple as it is, that the inexperienced person fails. A single slip may be fatal, and slips are constantly made. More-

infants' lives that it accomplishes in cutting out infectious diseases. (The writer wishes to record his indebtedness to Dr. J. P. Sedgwick, of Minneapolis, for much valuable information on this subject.)

[7] Once more we beg our readers not to think that, because building up the body cannot make it proof against infectious diseases, building up the body should be abandoned. To say that physical care of the body never made a Newton or a Shakespeare is not to say that no man need care for his physical welfare. The laws of physical health, even so little as we know of them, have many virtues. Because protection from infectious diseases is not one of them detracts no whit from any of the others.

[8] Tuberculosis and pneumonia are often held exceptions to this rule, but that they are exceptions is being questioned.

THE NEWEST PRACTICE 87

over, to guard against those infected persons *who are not recognized as such,* means that *all* discharges must be kept out of *all* mouths at *all* times,— a theoretically possible, but, to the vast majority of the work-a-day world, a practically wholly impossible, performance. If we give up in despair the hope of excluding *all* discharges from *all* mouths and attempt to teach the ordinary citizen to recognize infection so that he may avoid at least infected discharges, we shall be attempting to make of each citizen, man, woman, and child, a highly trained physician. To teach personal defense against infection is a great thing for those who have the opportunity to learn and the incentive to practice it. As a general method for abolishing infectious diseases it is quite hopeless; nevertheless, each citizen should have the chance to know at least the principles and these should be taught in every school in the land.

Those who believe that infectious disease should be warded off by specific immunization have some sure ground to go upon; but the scope of immunization is at present small. These are they who would build wolf-proof folds; but we do not know how to build folds which will be proof against all kinds of these wolves. It is true we know how to build a fold which is proof against smallpox, and that is vaccination. Also we have lately completed a fold proof against typhoid, which is antityphoid inoculation. But, alas, granting such folds are built, driving the sheep into them is a procedure forbidden to public health, except under martial law.

In vaccination and in antityphoid inoculation the old adage still applies: "First catch your sheep."

Those who believe in guarding routes of infection are those who would patrol the approaches to the sheep. This is at least a possible method, already established as of great value in some diseases. But a consideration of the following table shows that, like immunization, its scope is limited. Its scope is broader than that of immunization, but it is not broad enough to cover all infectious diseases.

If we tabulate the different infectious diseases occurring in the temperate zone on the basis of their chief routes of transmission we find that water, food, flies, and milk are the main public routes; the many private routes we group under contact; but not every route operates in every disease. Thus:

The Chief Infectious Diseases of the Temperate Zone classified by their Chief Routes of Infection

Typhoid fever (and other
   intestinal infections)
   are carried chiefly by ....water; food; flies; milk; contact.
Tuberculosis (human) [9] is
   carried chiefly by ....flies; [10] milk; contact.

[9] Bovine tuberculosis is of course derived chiefly from the milk of tuberculous cows. In many ways this disease is best separated for administrative purposes from human tuberculosis. The carriage of human tuberculosis in milk referred to in the table is that dependent on the infection of milk by tuberculous milk handlers.

[10] Insignificant.

THE NEWEST PRACTICE

Diphtheria, scarlet fever, measles, German measles, mumps, whooping-cough, smallpox, chickenpox are carried chiefly by......................milk; contact.
Syphilis, gonorrhea, trachoma, cerebro-spinal meningitis, leprosy are carried chiefly by ....contact

Hence water and food, as great public routes of community infections, carry only the intestinal infectious diseases. Flies, practically speaking, also carry this group only, the amount of tuberculosis carried by flies being small. Milk carries many infectious diseases, but contact alone carries all.

If we guard only water supplies against infection, we eliminate water-borne intestinal infections (this, so far as typhoid is concerned, would be perhaps one-third of the total typhoid in America). We leave untouched intestinal infections carried by food, flies, milk, and contact. Also we leave untouched *all other infectious diseases.*[11] If we guard food, as well as water, we eliminate such intestinal infections as are carried by food and water, but the fly, milk, and contact routes for these remain; so do *all routes* which carry *the other* infectious diseases.

[11] Hazen's theorem — that infected water supplies carry all the infectious diseases — is an unproved and much disputed hypothesis as yet.

If we eliminate flies also, fly typhoid and its congeners go, but milk and contact typhoid still remain with us. It is true that a slight effect on tuberculosis also might be noted, but nothing else is touched. If we guard milk supplies against infection,[12] we begin to make great strides, but *contact,* the great route of human tuberculosis and of all the other infectious diseases, including the intestinal, still will operate.

The fact is that while public water, food, fly, and milk infections parallel invasion by wolves *coming from without,* contact infection parallels the presence *amongst the sheep themselves,* of "wolves in sheep's clothing." Such wolves, because intermingled with the sheep, cannot possibly be eliminated by guarding the approaches.

If, then, the guarding of public routes can exclude only some of the infection, what remains?

The extermination of all the wolves — the abolition of the sources of infection.

If our modern wolf-hunters can find the undisguised wolves and even the wolves in sheep's clothing, *after* the sheep are slain, why cannot they find them also *before* the sheep are slain? If the very *sources* of infection (known cases, missed cases, and carriers) can-

[12] A great deal of the alleged milk supervision of to-day to prevent watering or to keep up the fat standard has no relation whatever to guarding milk against infection. Even the campaign for clean milk eliminates dirt chiefly. Unless especially conducted to prevent infection, it fails on this latter score completely. Most public health authorities now recommend heating even the "cleanest" milk as the only real safeguard.

THE NEWEST PRACTICE 91

not escape our epidemiologists armed with their modern principles, why wait for an epidemic before we go after them at all?

Turn again to the table and see that if we begin operations for control with water, we must move through food and flies and milk to contact before we have included all even of typhoid; and until we reach contact, we do not begin to touch the bulk of the other diseases at all. But if we begin with control of contact, we find that *the method which eliminates contact infection necessarily eliminates the other forms also.* That method when shorn of non-essentials is the supervision of *all* infectious persons.

THE NEW PROGRAM

To drop metaphors, the new program of official public health is the abolition of the infectious diseases.

The measures proposed for this purpose in progressive order of general efficiency, from lowest to highest, are —

1. The securing to each individual citizen continuously of his highest possible general physical health. Ideal as this is as an end in itself, it can have little effect on most infectious diseases, except indirectly during infancy, although it is acclaimed as a factor in reducing tuberculosis and pneumonia even in adults.

2. The securing to each individual citizen of instruction and training in the personal conduct which he must follow in order to avoid receiving into his body the dis-

charges of infected persons. This as a system is perfect, but the securing of the daily carrying out by every one of the personal conduct needed is a hopeless dream.

3. The securing to each individual of continuous specific immunization. Technically practical as yet only against smallpox and typhoid fever by inoculation, and in infancy against certain infections by breast-feeding, the scope of this procedure is very limited; and it must be remembered that the public have never yet adopted even smallpox immunization, except under compulsion, to an extent sufficient to abolish even this one disease.

These three measures place the abolition of infection directly upon the individual, as though, to abolish footpads, we should arm each citizen and train him in *jiu jitsu;* or as though, because of one free wolf, we should put five hundred sheep in armor. The three measures which follow place the abolition of infection directly upon a very small group of experts who deal directly with the infection itself. These three measures would put the one wolf in bonds, and let the five hundred sheep go free.

4. The physical supervision of the four great public routes of infection (public water supplies, public food supplies, flies, which are public property, and public milk supplies) to exclude all discharges from them. The principles are well understood, but, in practice, systematic application usually is lacking. (Physical supervision of such public and private surroundings as, by their effect on conduct, may bear on the operation

of the fifth and greatest route of all, i.e., contact, now more or less efficiently attempted in housing and settlement movements, is necessarily at present more a matter of education than of official action, especially where private surroundings are involved.)

5. The physical supervision of all *known* infectious cases to exclude their infected discharges from all routes. This, thoroughly done, would make a tremendous impression on infectious disease. But *known* cases form not more than half the total sources of infection.

6. *The sociological supervision of all infectious persons.* These are *the* sources of infectious diseases. Once found and supervised, infection from the human *must* stop *in toto*.

For the first three measures, education, demonstration, persuasion, are the things required; but also the abolition of carelessness, poverty, and the pressure of necessity. Knowledge alone is not enough; time and facilities to do with are needed also. To supply all these to every citizen, man, woman and child, is an ideal to be sought by every path; but an ideal that will take long years to realize.

For the second three we have principles and practice, precedent, authority, some law, and the hearty support of public opinion *in epidemics*. We need a few new laws. Chiefly we need proper organization and increased equipment; but, more than all, the hearty support of public opinion, *continuously,* not in epidemics only.

Of all these measures, the last is certainly the most inclusive; properly done, it excludes the need (so far as abolition of infectious diseases is concerned) of all the others. It is cheaper, simpler, easier, more direct and rapid than any other, and does not "interfere" with every citizen, in every act of daily life, indefinitely, for it deals with but one small class (infected persons), and only while infective; and it deals, even with them, merely to the extent of preventing the spread to others of their infected discharges.

CHAPTER IX

INDIVIDUAL DEFENSE

PUBLIC DEFENSE AND PRIVATE

The preceding chapter distinguished sharply those things necessary to *escape* existing chances of infection, which individuals *may* do, from those things necessary to *prevent* chances of infection from existing at all, which latter communities *must* do, if it be done at all, because individuals cannot.

The present chapter will outline the former, the individual's part in protecting himself. As already indicated, these individual efforts may be made in three directions:

1. To secure high general physical health.
2. To secure specific immunity to specific diseases.
3. To avoid disease, especially infectious disease.

Efforts made in the first direction aim to build up and make palaces of the bodies in which we dwell and which, too often, are mere hovels; but, alas, the non-fireproof palace burns as easily as the non-fireproof hovel. It is futile to seek the physical advancement of the race in order *to abolish disease*. We should seek the abolition of disease in order *to physically advance the race.*[1]

THE PREVENTABILITY OF THE "PREVENTABLE" DISEASES

True, we should not await the abolition of disease before seeking general physical advancement, but, unfortunately for the achievement of very much real progress

[1] No greater fallacy burdens public health advance than the idea that high health protects against infection. Every health officer scouts this idea when it is presented to him by an antivaccinationist to show that vaccination is unnecessary — scouts it when it is offered as an excuse for neglecting quarantine — scouts it when father, mother, nurse, wife, husband urge it as a reason why he or she, untrained in self-protection, should brave infection at the side of a loved one. Yet almost every health officer will urge it in his next bulletin or in his next address! The statement that high health is an efficient protection against infection is either true or not true. When athletes, soldiers in the pink of condition, lumbermen, fail to succumb to syphilis, gonorrhea, typhoid, pneumonia, it will be time to consider high health as a possible reason for their escape. Until that time this wretched quibble should be abandoned by all who hope to teach the truth according to the evidence.

The Agricultural colleges and experiment stations, dealing with the physical development of stock animals to the highest point, have found that such high physical development does not prevent or minimize infection. It is high grade stock, rather than scrub, which suffers infections. Immunity to certain diseases has been secured by careful breeding amongst plants (rustless wheat for instance), but not amongst animals to any practical extent. (Permission to quote their names in support of this footnote has been granted by Dean A. F. Woods of the University of Minnesota Agricultural Department, and by **Principal F. C. Harrison** of the MacDonald College, Quebec.)

INDIVIDUAL DEFENSE

in this line, we know as yet few practicable rules of general application, except for infants, to achieve such physical advancement. Far better than how to secure high physical health we know how to avoid disease, at least, how to avoid certain diseases. A few of these are non-infectious environmental diseases, like scurvy and miner's elbow; and the non-infectious poisonings, like those from lead, arsenic, phosphorus, alcohol, and illuminating gas. These diseases depend upon readily recognized mechanical or physical surroundings. A change of diet in scurvy or of position in miner's elbow; stopping leaks in pipes for illuminating gas poisoning; refusal to admit the other poisons to the body — and all are abolished. But after all, these non-infectious poisons furnish but 1 in 1,000 of all deaths, except in infancy, where non-infectious intestinal poisonings probably furnish a large proportion.

On the other hand, the poisonings which are infectious, i.e., the infectious diseases, furnish more than one-sixth of all the deaths, and about one-half of these deaths are from but one infectious disease, namely, consumption. Like the chemical poisonings,— lead, arsenic, etc.,— the infectious diseases depend on noxious materials that enter the body. But, unlike lead, arsenic, etc., the poisons which produce the infectious diseases are associated, not with a few well-known material *surroundings* and inanimate *things,* but with the living activities of many, often unknown, *persons.*

The little we know of how to achieve high health, and

98   THE NEW PUBLIC HEALTH

the much more we know of how to avoid disease, should be taught our many million citizens. This huge task requires a mechanism so huge that only our huge public school system can accomplish it.[2]

Efforts in the second direction (for specific immunization) aim to "fireproof" our bodies against disease, whether those bodies be "palaces" or "hovels." But such fireproofing can as yet be done only against smallpox and typhoid fever.[3]

Also, just as the general public will not fireproof literal houses against literal fire, despite large fire losses every year, so the general public will not fireproof their bodies against infection, even against smallpox. One

[2] It is often said that practicing physicians should teach health to the public. In one sense this is true. Physicians represent medicine, and medicine deals with disease, its cure and its prevention. But practicing engineers might as well be drafted to teach geometry as practicing physicians to teach personal hygiene. Physicians dealing with their own patients, or even lecturing or writing on these subjects, do much good. Such work, however, is but a drop in the bucket, reaching only a fraction of the public and generally just that fraction which needs it least. There are over 100,000 practicing physicians in America. They have not time, training, organization, or authority for the sort of teaching that will really reach all citizens; the public school system has all four, and nearly a million teachers to do it with.

Medicine must furnish the facts that are to be taught, but it is quite impossible that practising physicians should do the teaching.

[3] The immunity possible against diphtheria through protective doses of diphtheria antitoxin, is too short-lived for general continuous application to all citizens.

hundred years of vaccination has left us with only 30 per cent. of children under 16 years of age protected against smallpox. We shall be lucky if 10 years of antityphoid inoculation finds us with 10 per cent. of adults protected against typhoid. In the absence of compulsory laws, rigorously enforced, immunization must remain a task of systematic education, reaching every one, and this task also only the public school system can properly perform.

Efforts in the third direction aim to shut out all poisons, including all infections, from all bodies, whether these bodies be palaces or hovels, on the principle that as no dwelling, palace or hovel, can burn if fire do not reach it, so our bodies, good, bad, or indifferent, cannot be destroyed by disease if the causes of disease be shut out from them. To abolish literal fire from literal dwellings is impracticable, for fire is too useful for such abolition. Disease serves no useful purpose, and its abolition is the only reasonable goal.

The exclusion of the poisons of disease, infectious or non-infectious, from the body, is the most successful preventive measure we have at present against most diseases that are preventable at all. The methods should be taught to every citizen; and for this again the public school system alone is able. Public health experts must supply the facts; it is quite impossible that they should do the teaching.[4]

[4] Of each 1,000 school children 450 leave school at the end of the 6th grade work, 450 leave at the end of the 8th grade. The

"DODGING INFECTION"

"Dodging infection" rests on simple principles, already outlined. The one essential is to exclude from entrance to the body, matter from infectious bodies, i.e., in briefest practical form, to *exclude from the body, usually from the mouth, the infected discharges of others.*[5]

To do this requires, first, the ability to recognize infectious persons; and, second, the skill to avoid their discharges. But we cannot teach the general public, half of them children, to recognize infectious persons. If, then, we broaden the rule and teach avoidance of discharges of all sick persons, whether infectious or not, we ignore those persons who are infectious without being sick. Hence, for the non-medical citizen, the rule must run: Exclude *all* discharges of *all* persons from *all*

remaining 100 enter the high school; but only 50 graduate. Ten out of the thousand enter the University; 5 graduate. We now teach in the earlier grades theoretical anatomy and theoretical physiology, intending thus to form foundations for later practical information. Since 90 per cent. of children leave at or before the 8th grade, this 90 per cent. receive the theoretical information only; they never learn its practical use at all.

This system needs inversion. We should teach the practical parts of hygiene and of avoidance of disease to the 100 per cent. of children, i.e., not later than the 6th grade, leaving the theoretical parts for the 10 per cent. that take the higher courses.

[5] Plague, malaria, yellow fever, typhus are, in most cases, the results of bites of insects infected from infectious bodies. The principle is the same although the modes of transmission differ.

INDIVIDUAL DEFENSE 101

bodies, especially the mouth. But this is by no means so easy as it sounds.

CONTACT-INFECTION

The mouth-discharges of our associates are constantly entering our bodies in the form of mouth-spray, of sputum, and of smears on various things, but *chiefly by smears on hands*.

Mouth-spray consists of tiny, often microscopic, drops of liquid from the mouth, thrown out in sneezing, coughing, shouting, singing, and speaking, but not in quiet breathing. The larger ones can be seen, if watched for, and they can be felt falling upon the face during close face-to-face conversations. Talk, or sing, or shout, or cough, or sneeze against a mirror two feet distant, and count the drops that strike it. Then picture to yourself what happens at " teas " and " sociables "; at meals, with lively conversation going on; at school; at church. Think also of what happens when cooks or waiters talk while preparing food, cough while laying tables, or sneeze while wiping dishes.

This distribution of mouth-spray cannot be *prevented* unless all wear masks, as modern surgeons do when operating.

But the intaking of mouth-spray may be *avoided somewhat* by avoiding close face-to-face conversations, as by sitting side by side or far apart; its distribution to others by coughing or sneezing always into a handkerchief, etc. Often, of course, the cough or sneeze comes too quickly or the hands are already full. It is true that the head may be turned aside; but often this spares the person in front at the expense of others, and, while coughing or sneezing into the hand prevents the mouth-spray from flying wide, the spray goes to the hand and the hand itself passes it on to other persons later.

There is no practical method of avoiding all mouth-spray of associates, except not to have associates; but the amount of exchange may be diminished by the above precautions.

Sputum, through the spitting habit, falls upon floors, steps, sidewalks. That these deposits dry and blow about as dust is the least of the dangers, especially out of doors, for sunlight and drying disable most disease germs. Sputum follows a much more important route leading to mouths, and this route is followed, not when the sputum has become dry and dusty, but while it is still fresh and moist,— while disease germs which may be in it are still living. This route is by way of shoes, directly into houses. There, wiped off on carpets, it awaits the creeping baby; it smears itself on the baby's fingers; and they carry it directly into his mouth. Also, the owner of the shoes uses his fingers in removing shoes, and then, too often, the owner's fingers, just like the baby's, enter the mouth unwashed. The value of anti-spitting ordinances thus becomes apparent.

But, after all, hands are the great route of exchange, and hands furnish the great route for bladder,

INDIVIDUAL DEFENSE 103

bowel and other discharges, as well as for nose and mouth.[6]

From birth to death those universal tools, our hands, go to our mouths incessantly; from birth to death we use them for every other purpose also. Hands encounter all the discharges of the body many times a day; and if not scrupulously washed on every such occasion, they carry these discharges to everything they touch, including other hands, which go to other mouths. The very handkerchiefs we advocate to cough or sneeze or blow our noses into, transfer these same discharges to our fingers, the next time that we use them.[7] Then we shake hands with others, or feel the baby's new tooth.

Visits to toilets, unless followed at once by careful hand-washing, mean similar transfer of the toilet discharges as well, particularly amongst children, who, remember, form nearly half the population.

The common drinking-cup and the common drinking-pail are bad because they help to exchange mouth-discharges; the roller-towel is worse, especially when used for *half-washed* hands, because then it helps to exchange *all* the bodily discharges; but the *unwashed* hands themselves are worst of all, because the discharges they carry are undiluted and fresh and moist and warm. When

[6] Hands do not carry infectious diseases only. They are the chief routes by which lead is carried to mouths in lead-poisoning, and are also an important factor in phosphorus poisoning.

[7] It has been suggested that the left hand should be used for handkerchiefs, thus leaving the right hand clean so far as these discharges are concerned.

strangers enter a household, they add, through mouth-spray and hands, their discharges to the general household stock; and, in this way, harvesting help, threshing crews, etc., introduce infectious disease into numerous rural families and communities every year.

Within the purview of the private citizen at home, discharges are also exchanged somewhat through *things* soiled by mouth-spray and hands, as well as directly. Thus are contaminated dishes in laying the table, bread, cake, etc., also pillow-cases and sheets which are soiled by mouth or other discharges from the body. The list of the things which *may* carry such discharges is too long for itemizing here; but, in general, such *things* do not form really very important routes of transfer, except when the discharges are considerable in quantity and while the discharges are fresh and moist. Once dried on clothing, mouth-spray, for instance, is not readily set free, and when it is dry, infection, if present, dies out with fair rapidity. Just as the main public routes of discharges from the community to the family are public water supplies, public food supplies, public milk supplies, and public outdoor flies, so the main private routes within the family, apart from mouth-spray, sputum, and hands, are private water supplies, private food supplies, private milk supplies, and private indoor flies. Public supplies may or may not bring discharges with them to the family; once they enter the family, they pretty surely receive the family discharges from the family itself. So also with the private sup-

INDIVIDUAL DEFENSE 105

plies of the same things; the family well may or may not be dosed with the family discharges; the family drinking-pail or pitcher almost always is; the family cow may or may not contribute discharges to the family milk-pail, but the family milker practically always does;[8] and later, within the family, the family milk-pitcher receives the family mouth-spray. The family food, before and even after cooking, is subject to similar contamination. The family flies moving from the outdoor toilet, unless it be fly-proof, or from indoor spittoons or slops to food, aid in the same exchange.[9]

To know these dangers means half the battle won.

[8] If a milker talks or sings or coughs or sneezes, using a wide mouth pail, his mouth discharges enter the milk. If he milks with unwashed hands, *all* his discharges enter the milk also.

[9] A curious perversity of human nature makes us attach undue importance to many possible but unimportant routes of discharges, like telephone-receivers, dirty money, the licking of postage stamps, etc., while we neglect the commonplace, really important routes, acting daily and everywhere, above outlined.

An example of the same thing is seen in the great anxiety expressed concerning meat as a route of infection. It seems to be remembered but seldom that meat is almost always cooked, i.e., it almost always automatically receives the very treatment we solicitously prescribe for blocking infection through milk and through water. Meat-inspection is wholly proper, to secure good meat, and to prevent the robbing of the consumer's pocket and the consumer's stomach. But all the meat-inspection in the world could not reduce our ordinary infectious diseases by one-tenth of 1 per cent. Meat, as food, especially cold meat, often carries the family discharges, but disease in, or discharges attached to, meat from its sources outside the family, are in most cases destroyed by cooking.

Against infection of public routes,— public water supplies, public food supplies, public outdoor flies, and public milk supplies,— the private citizen should not need precautions, for these the community itself should guard. But if he need them, the private citizen has against such public routes two powerful weapons: (a) exclusion from his premises of the infected material, and (b) cooking. Foods are, of course, usually cooked, even in ordinary life; water may be boiled, milk heated, and if flies cannot be excluded, the food they contaminate can be rejected or cooked again.

The public routes of infection are not difficult for the citizen to guard against, however wearisome that guarding may be; the real difficulty is with the private routes, those routes of contact that carry infection within the family and also within the school, the office, the workshop, the factory. We, individually or collectively, may abolish in time the common drinking-cup and common roller-towel, but no one can ever abolish mouth-spray or hands throughout the race.[10]

It is true that by education [11] we may greatly affect

[10] One hundred million mouths, served by 200,000,000 hands, receive 300,000,000 meals in America daily. But these hands are not as important as are the hands that handle the meals in preparation; moreover, hands go to mouths far more often between meals than during them.

[11] The following rules prepared for use in the public schools at the request of County Superintendent Geo. S. Selke, Benton County, Minnesota, indicate the main points to be taught concerning protection from infectious diseases in the schools. They indicate also pretty closely what can be done in the home and for

INDIVIDUAL DEFENSE 107

personal conduct, but to leave the abolition of infection in ordinary life to the personal conduct of all sorts of people, half of them children, would be as wise as to

this reason they are inserted here. (Now printed and distributed to Minnesota Schools by the State Department of Education.)

Placard for Schools

The germs of infectious diseases are in the discharges of infectious persons. Infectious diseases are "caught" from infectious persons simply by taking into the mouth some portion, usually very small, of their infected discharges.

The Great Rules of Prevention in Schools

1. Exclude from school all infectious persons, thus excluding all infectious discharges.

2. Since infectious persons may enter school at times despite the greatest vigilance, restrict, so far as possible, the scattering of any discharge of any person at any time in school. (This will also train the children to restrict their discharges out of school and in after-life.)

a. Mouth discharges are transferred directly to and taken directly from drinking-cups, towels, pencils, chewing-gum, whistles, etc. Mouth, nose, bladder, and bowel discharges are transferred directly to hands many times daily. Hands go to mouths many times daily; therefore —

Provide individual drinking-cups, individual towels, individual pencils, individual modeling-clay, individual modeling-sand, etc. (There should be a sign in every school, "Wash your hands after every visit to a toilet.")

b. Sputum (spit) or other discharges, deposited on floors, sidewalks, etc., are picked up by shoes and so carried into homes. When handling shoes (putting on, taking off, etc.), discharges are transferred to hands, which go to mouths, or touch things that go to mouths. Therefore —

Avoid depositing discharges,— sputum, etc.,— on floors, sidewalks, or elsewhere where other people may step on them.

trust the destruction of infection in a water-borne typhoid outbreak to the boiling of the water by private citizens.

c. Mouth-spray is thrown out in talking, singing, coughing, sneezing, etc., therefore —
Avoid throwing mouth-spray into other people's faces by avoiding close face-to-face conversation, face-to-face recitations, face-to-face singing-exercises, etc. Cough, sneeze, etc., into a handkerchief always.

d. The air of a schoolroom in use necessarily receives mouth-spray into it in talking, reciting, etc.

e. Bladder and bowel discharges are carried by flies when flies can get at them. During early autumn and late spring or summer sessions, flies may carry these discharges from toilets to children's lunches, etc., therefore —
Make toilet-vaults fly-proof. Provide springs or weights to automatically close toilet-doors, and fly-screens for toilet-windows.

f. Three things destroy comfort and success in school work: Temperature too high; Atmosphere too dry; Air not in motion. Also, no child can work well in a poorly lighted room; but do not imagine that good lighting, good heating, and good ventilation will prevent spread of infection if infectious persons gain entrance. No school is a sanitary school if the children exchange their discharges without restriction; but only those schools where infectious persons are watched for and excluded are safe schools, therefore —
Note daily the general state of health of each child. No child who shows any decided change from the usual for that child, especially fever, headache, sore throat, stomach-ache, or general dumpishness, should attend school until seen by a physician. This rule permits early detection of infectious children. It also excludes children who should be excluded for their own good, even if non-infectious.

g. Children showing defective vision, hearing, breathing, etc., should be referred to the principal, superintendent, or school board for action.

All health officers know that adults in large proportion *will not,* and many children *cannot,* boil the water. Moreover, the law (in Minnesota) now recognizes that the community has no right to supply water of such a kind that the consumer must protect himself against it. This principle should be extended, so that the community is held responsible for infection carried by any public route,— food, milk, or flies,— as well as by public water. Some day the equally logical step should follow,— the holding of the community responsible for *all* infectious diseases, by *whatever* routes they travel, including contact. The community, thanks to modern science, can abolish the sources of all infectious diseases; and once the sources are abolished, the diseases, being non-existent, *cannot* travel by any route, even by contact.

The simple fact is, that the private citizen in his own home can protect himself against public routes of discharges as just outlined and from the family discharges to some extent; but the moment he leaves home and enters into relations with the general public, his individual control is at an end. He cannot guard, generally he cannot even ascertain, the sources or routes of the water, milk, food, or flies he must encounter. Above all, he cannot guard the sources or routes of the discharges furnished by the persons he necessarily meets. His children go to school, compelled directly by the law to do so, and there they share discharges which no personal defense through conduct can wholly avoid. He goes himself to work, compelled indirectly by the law to do so, and there he shares discharges which he can little or not at all control. Only the community can *exclude* infection from the public routes of discharges, water, milk, food, and flies; but also only the community can *exclude* infection from the private routes of discharges grouped under " contact "; for only the community can exercise such control over those already infected as to prevent them distributing their infection.

Of course, the exchange of discharges already outlined, however inevitable, is harmless unless and until infected discharges enter into the exchange. The chances of encountering infected discharges can be approximated somewhat from the supposition that daily there goes at large, unknown, say one infective person in each 500 of the population. Hence, he who would defend himself from infection by his habitual personal conduct toward his associates must avoid the harmless discharges of 499 uninfected persons in order to avoid the harmful discharges of one unknown infected person. (This estimate is necessarily a guess, and it does not include the venereal infections.)

The great weakness of the personal defense through conduct is this: The precise moment when it is most needed is the precise moment when it generally fails. In the first place, the mouth-spray of the ordinary well person is not half so abundant or so widely scattered as that of the case of tuberculosis, of measles, of whooping-cough, or of influenza, for these are just the diseases

INDIVIDUAL DEFENSE 111

in which coughing and sneezing are prominent symptoms. The bowel-discharges of the ordinary well person are not half as likely to be disseminated as those of the typhoid or dysentery case, for these are just the diseases in which frequent, abundant liquid stools, often involuntary, occur. Again, the discharges of the well person are handled chiefly by that well person himself; the discharges of the sick must often be handled by associates unused to performing such services for others. Finally, exactly as green troops forget under fire all their parade-ground drill, trip over their own feet, and fire into the ground or at the sun, so the citizen, however carefully he may have practiced a well-thought-out system of avoiding discharges in ordinary life, goes all to pieces in the flurry when his child develops, say, scarlet fever. Of course, it is true that untried troops soon recover their parade-ground drill, even in the face of the enemy; but they cannot do what seasoned troops can do, and the non-medical citizen can seldom protect himself in the face of infection as the trained contagious-disease nurse does, the physician, or the epidemiologist. Nevertheless, if he has previously known, and practiced even crudely, the necessary precautions,[12] he is in a much better position to defend himself.

[12] It is a fatal fallacy to believe in " general cleanliness " as a defense against infection. It is not the " general cleanliness " of surroundings that prevents infectious diseases; it is the " *specific* cleanliness " of freedom from infected discharges. Scrubbed floors, bright pans, neatness, and order do not necessarily involve, usually do not imply, hands free of discharges; they

SUMMARY

The whole subject of public health divides itself into —
1. Securing high physical development and efficiency.
2. Avoiding disease.

Of the former we know little of practical application to the general population except in infancy.

Of the latter we know much of cure, but little of prevention, except in the environmental diseases, in the poisonings, as from lead, arsenic, alcohol, etc., and especially in the infectious diseases.

Defense against environmental diseases and the noninfectious poisonings is largely a matter of trade conditions and of avoiding dangerous, but known, nonliving things and therefore largely of legislation, inspection, and conduct. Against infectious diseases, the sources being infected persons, defense is essentially a matter of precautions against those persons. The prime difficulty is the recognition of those persons. If they are not recognized, the defense becomes a matter of guarding against *all* persons.

Defense against infection may be divided into individual and community defense.

Infectious diseases are carried by four main public

cannot stop mouth-spray. A gorgeous uniform no more shows ability to shoot than does "general cleanliness" show ability to avoid infection. It is not visible dirt that hurts,— mud, ashes, coal-dust,— but the usually invisible discharges in mouth-spray and on hands, and even these only when laden with infection.

INDIVIDUAL DEFENSE 113

routes — water, food, flies, and milk; and by a fifth private route, contact. By cooking *all* alimentary supplies before eating them, the public routes may be guarded at the consumers' end, but public opinion and, in the matter of water supplies, the law (in Minnesota), rightly demand the transfer of this burden of protection to the producer.

The private routes of contact can be guarded by the individual also, but only by a ritual so elaborate and covering so general a field that it does not adequately meet the ordinary conditions of the ordinary life of the ordinary citizen, especially of hard-working fathers, hard-driven mothers and young children. Contagious-disease experts, with long, patient training and when dealing with known infected individuals, generally succeed; the ordinary untrained citizen must very often fail.

Notwithstanding that the community can and should assume the prevention of contact-infection (by excluding infection from the community entirely), in addition to the care, now very general, of the four public routes, the methods of personal defense should be well known to all; and there exists no means of teaching them comparable at all with the great public school system, for that, and that alone, reaches the citizens personally and in detail. There, in simple language, all that is useful can be readily taught, and it must be taught in the sixth grade, or earlier, to reach the population as a whole.

CHAPTER X

COMMUNITY DEFENSE

THE PUBLIC HEALTH ENGINEER

The preceding chapter indicated the lines of personal defense against infectious disease which are available to the private citizen for his own protection through his own efforts.

The present and succeeding chapters will deal with community defense,— those operations which, if properly conducted by communities for the good of all, would make unnecessary the burdensome efforts of individuals to protect themselves.

The three great community measures for the abolition of infectious disease have been listed in increasing order of efficiency as —

1. The protection of all public routes of infection, public water supplies, public food supplies, public milk supplies, and public flies. This is now done in some places to some extent. Usually it is but half done, chiefly for lack of proper understanding of what are real protective measures, or of proper organization for their execution; too often, also for lack of proper men to carry them out.

COMMUNITY DEFENSE

2. The physical supervision of *known* cases of infectious diseases. This also is often now attempted. Indeed it is, on paper, the most developed of all. But its efficiency is cut down by lack of reporting, concealing of cases from and sometimes, alas, by physicians, etc., and especially by lack of sufficient trained experts in epidemiology to do the close-to-the-ground daily work.

3. The sociological supervision of all infectious persons, already outlined in previous articles.

The first of these items is dealt with here.

For the protection of the public routes of infection three things are needed: proper physical construction, to exclude infection; proper physical operation, to maintain this exclusion; and the supervision of the human factor,—" the man behind the gun." A locomotive may be built perfectly and be kept in perfect running order; but the locomotive engineer himself is still the soul of the machine. Perfect physical equipment and perfect physical maintenance of public utilities related to the spread of disease, are enormously important, yet they are less important than the men who are to be in actual control of the actual operations. No better illustration of this can be offered than the fact that the milk supply from tested highbred cows, palatially housed, scrubbed, and vacuum-cleaned, has many times carried disease and death to the customers, because some one man engaged in handling the milk conveyed infection to it by the intimate personal contact which no organization or mechanism can wholly avoid.

Some of the worst water epidemics we have ever had were due to the human factor failing at the critical moment. This failure of the human factor, which is a commonplace in accidents by rail or boat, applies equally to all branches of public health, although the usual belief is that almost any person is good enough to conduct public health work.

The reason for this commonly accepted belief is probably that public health work for the prevention of disease, or for the general physical advancement of the race, is often confused with certain measures which make merely for ease or comfort; and it is human nature to look down upon those whose services minister to our comfort. We forget that by our slaves we rise and by our slaves we fall. Too often they and their procedures are neglected so long as comfort and convenience are supplied by them without too much trouble to those who enjoy the fruits of their labor.

To define public health engineering in the light of the new public health principles, it must be defined as such work as deals through the physical construction and operation of physical surroundings and mechanisms with (a) the prevention of disease or (b) with the advancement of physical bodily welfare. If we include also, as is sometimes done, all such operations as conduce, however indirectly, to any kind of "racial advancement," we must add all engineering works, architecture, street paving, acoustic properties of public buildings, the size of doorways, fire-escapes, bridges,

COMMUNITY DEFENSE 117

railways, and every other form of modern artificial surroundings, and with them their corollaries, noise, dust, the smoke nuisance, etc.

The line between true sanitary measures and those for securing mere comfort or convenience must be drawn somewhere, and it must be remembered that all " racial advances " are by no means advancements of public health. The railroads are of great sociological importance to the race, but they often carry disease faster or further than it would have traveled otherwise. Every advance which leads to greater prosperity leads also to more intermingling of people and to wider social relations and so involves a wider exchange of bodily discharges. The installation of a public water supply system adds great comfort, convenience, decency, and physical welfare, but it also provides a route of infection theretofore non-existing, which leads directly into every home. If you put all your eggs into one such basket, you must *watch that basket.* A sewerage system, by getting rid of outdoor toilets, greatly conduces to decency, comfort, and cleanliness, and even obviates one danger of disease (carriage of toilet discharges by flies from the outdoor closet); but it also concentrates all those discharges into one foul union and the disposal of this often endangers other communities, and there is no real social advance in transferring the burden of infectious disease from one community to another by passing the sewage on from one water supply to another. Hence the true province of the Public Health

Engineer is not the mere advocacy and construction of great engineering enterprises, but, rather, the supervision of the construction of such, to see that the public health harm they may do, if the public health view be neglected, is properly avoided, so far as physical construction or operation may avoid it.

The Public Health Engineer is not therefore, or, rather, should not be, merely what the popular imagination makes him, a man of sewer pipes and concrete; of water-meters, manholes, and pumps. The New Public Health Engineer will be a man keen of eye to see those features in all community construction work which may conduce to greater exchange of discharges, a man who knows *just* what is needed for prevention of disease in such ways, and therefore can both provide adequate precautions and at the same time avoid unnecessary or excessive ones. The civil engineer has been defined as he who can do for $1.00 what any fool can do for $4.00. He is a physical economist. He insists on physical safety, but *within that limit* knows best how to achieve the needed safety without undue expenditure. The Public Health Engineer, dealing with water supplies, sewage disposal, etc., does just this thing. He guarantees sanitary safety, and *within that limit* he guarantees it for less money than the ordinary builder. Any keen student of infectious diseases can generally see the grosser faults in a supply which permit infection. The Public Health Engineer is a specialist. He sees these faults very much more quickly and surely; if

COMMUNITY DEFENSE 119

they are intricate he has the skill and knowledge to disentangle them; and when he finds them, he knows how to correct them.

The Public Health Engineer is, or should be, much more than this, however. He is the only public health worker whose initial professional training necessarily makes of him a business man, in the sense of an administrator of operations on schedule time, and with economy of labor and expense. Those physicians who make good administrators in this sense do so because they learn it in administration, not because of initial professional training. This training of the Public Health Engineer makes him also the best man to supervise maintenance of public utilities, as well as to construct and equip them. Further, the absence of training in mechanisms and machinery so prominent in the training of most health officials, makes of the Public Health Engineer the only public health man who can deal properly with the many mechanical devices for modern handling of the public routes of infection, on the perfection of which many lives often depend. The hypochlorite plant, the mechanical filter, the pasteurizing device are machines. However well a physician may understand the underlying biological principles, he cannot figure the pitch of a cog-wheel or find the reason of the filter "loss of head" without infinite and wasteful effort, if at all.

The Public Health Engineer is in public health what the surgeon is in medicine, the "man of his hands,"—

the actual operator. Whatever the physician may discover as surgically necessary to be done, it is the surgeon who must bring his skill and knowledge to bear upon the doing of it. So, although the epidemiologist, the vital statistician, the laboratory man must usually determine the sources and routes of disease, it is the Public Health Engineer to whom all must turn wherever and whenever those sources or routes are to be put out of action by physical construction or mechanical device, or when economic maladministration of public utilities is the real basis of the trouble, rather than a physical condition.

The Public Health Engineer is not, however, as a rule, a man of a biological turn of mind. He generally takes vital statistics too seriously and, lacking medical knowledge, interprets vital statistics too mechanically. His own units of weight, volume, and measurement are fixed and definite. He has not learned to scan the unfamiliar units of disease, each by itself; nor is it likely that as a class engineers ever will. The spectacle of an engineer advising on a strictly medical problem is only less sad, if less sad at all, than that of a medical man advising on a strictly engineering problem. It is by co-operation of these two, each perfect in his own field, but aiding the other with real understanding of the other's problem, that well-balanced, sane advance is made.

So far as the five great routes are concerned,— water, food, milk, flies, and contact,— the engineer has as yet

COMMUNITY DEFENSE 121

found his chief field in dealing with water supplies. Even sewage disposal, so far as it is a sanitary problem, has as yet been chiefly considered in relation to the purity of water. But in the future the engineer must also deal with milk supplies, their production, transportation, pasteurization, disinfection; with the great fly problem and its chief corollary, the safe disposal of human excreta, as well as its minor corollaries, garbage and manure removal. Finally, perhaps chiefly, he must deal with the great sociological factors on which rests contact infection in public meeting-places,— the factory, the shop, the church, the theater, the school, even the tenement and the private home. Above all, the great engineer of the future is he who will see with trained analytical mind and act with trained administrative ability in organizing or re-organizing not one but a dozen of the many factors in the modern complex of society, along lines which shall in themselves redistribute concentrated forces now too closely interwoven for mutual good.

But there must be more public health in engineering rather than more engineering in public health. This little book will have failed wholly in pointing out the real essential inside truth of public health progress if it leaves any implication that infectious diseases can be abolished through any physical or mechanical means. The great engineering operations of the day have an importance to mankind much greater in sociological and economic lines than in public health. But the public health end must not be neglected, even though we recognize that it can never be the great end of engineering, because no mere guarding of such *routes* of infection can abolish disease, and, if it could, there are far more direct, drastic, and simple measures to be enforced in other directions than in the protection of public utilities. Great engineering works are not essential to the abolition of infectious diseases, but great engineering works should be so conducted as to secure what reduction in such diseases they may. The ultimate abolition of infectious diseases rests with the supervision of the infectious individual, and no mere adjustment of surroundings practical for the race, can so affect his conduct as to compel that conduct along proper lines. But the public health engineer through housing, organization, and the proper construction and supervision of public utilities, can so design the lines of least resistance that the public, who generally follow these lines, will find them plain and smooth, but hedged about with iron walls of safety.

SUMMARY

It is a complete misnomer to designate as a sanitary engineer him who merely narrows his attention from the principles and practice of engineering in general to the application of these principles for the purpose of constructing water supplies, sewage-disposal systems, rendering of garbage, etc.

A man is not a sanitary engineer because he can lay

COMMUNITY DEFENSE 123

down sewer pipe any more than a man is an artist because he can lay on paint. The Public Health Engineer in the true sense is he who has acquired so wide a view of modern life, of its mechanisms, and of the physical side of man's environments, that he can see and act through them for man's physical protection, not merely from accident but also from disease. He does not just build sewers. When he builds them, he builds them as part of the great fabric of modern life. His plans are not merely so many feet of pipe, at such a price per foot; they are adaptations and applications of great fundamental laws to the physical advancement of mankind.

CHAPTER XI

COMMUNITY DEFENSE

THE PUBLIC-HEALTH LABORATORY

THE previous chapter discussed the relation of the Public Health engineer to the protection of man from disease, through the construction, operation, and direction of those public utilities already proved to be, at times, *routes* of infection.

Some day, when we have really determined the conditions which truly promote physical well-being, as distinguished from those which merely secure escape from disease, the Public Health engineer will find larger functions in a wider field, the supervision of the whole material surroundings of man.

The present chapter attempts to set forth the relation of the Public Health laboratory man to the same two divisions,— to the promotion of high health, on the one hand, and to the prevention of disease, on the other. Like the Public Health engineer, the Public Health laboratory man can as yet contribute but little to the former, and for the same reason, i.e., because so little is really known about it. Like the Public Health engineer, the Public Health laboratory man deals with the

COMMUNITY DEFENSE 125

prevention of disease, and chiefly with the prevention of the infectious diseases. Again, like the engineer, the laboratory man deals in part with *routes* of diseases, with those public utilities which at times form highways for the exchange of infected, and uninfected, bodily discharges. But, unlike the engineer, his work is not confined to *routes*.

The Public Health laboratory man, like the epidemiologist, deals also with *sources,* i.e., with the infected person. In some ways he goes further than the epidemiologist, for he deals with the infected discharges themselves, rather than with the person who discharges them; and, not stopping even there, he deals with, in those discharges, the very principles of disease itself,—the individual little particles of living matter whose activities in the human system produce so much trouble for us all.

This dealing intimately with the ultimate causes of disease is a fascinating, dangerous, peculiar life-work, an actual herding, and handling of the very essences of the dreaded plagues of old. What would not the ancient philosophers and sages have given for one glimpse of a modern Public Health laboratory where matter-of-fact men handle, in their daily matter-of-fact routine, diphtheria plants, typhoid plants, tuberculosis plants, etc., quite as a student farmer handles potatoes or corn?

Because the little plants, or animals that produce many of our common diseases are as yet not actually known, for instance those of scarlet fever, measles, and smallpox, to name only three, the Public Health laboratory man's chief daily duties lie with those diseases the germs of which are known, and therefore chiefly with the germs of typhoid, diphtheria, and tuberculosis. These furnish the bulk of his work. His chief services to mankind, in the temperate zone at least, consist in the aid he gives in recognizing those persons who are infected with one of these three germs without showing conclusive, perhaps any, symptoms of their presence. True, he can and does perform like services in other diseases whose germs are known — such as anthrax, bubonic plague, cholera, glanders, leprosy, etc.; but these are so rare as to form only a flavoring for his daily grist. In the venereal diseases, also, the biological causes are known and can be recognized, but the laboratory man must await the development of the growing public demand for the handling of these diseases on a par with other infections, the taking up of these great subjects by legislative and executive authorities. Until that time comes the laboratory man can proclaim his own readiness and point to the road, but he can do little more.[1]

With the *routes* of infection,— water, flies, food, milk, and contact,— the laboratory man has much to do, but, again and for similar reasons, he deals with these routes, in the temperate zone, chiefly when typhoid,

[1] Laboratory tests for syphilis and gonorrhea are becoming recognized of late as Public Health laboratory duties. (See New York Health Department and others.)

diphtheria, or tuberculosis are involved. His functions in all this work are chiefly analytic, i.e., to find the particular water, or milk, or food which may be dangerous; sometimes to detect, if he may, the presence in them of the deadly germ itself.

Unfortunately, the laboratory, for reasons already offered in a different connection, can rarely find the germs of disease in water, food, milk, or flies. They live so short a life outside of the human, or animal, bodies which form their natural growing-grounds that the laboratory man seldom encounters them except in the body. As a general thing, long before a "sample" of water, etc., arrives at the laboratory, the disease germs it may once have held are dead or so outgrown by others that the best laboratory methods must necessarily fail to find them.

So little is this understood that one of the almost daily happenings in every laboratory is the receipt of water, or milk, or food (flies, fortunately, are not often sent, as yet) from laymen, even from physicians, with the request that they be searched for typhoid or diphtheria germs.

But consider! Before a given water supply has attention called to it as a source of typhoid fever, typhoid fever cases usually must have developed from it. Now, typhoid fever is a disease which does not develop even its very first symptoms, until, on an average, two weeks have elapsed after the germs first entered the body from the water supply. Usually, another week passes before the physician is called and perhaps another week, more often two or three, before the sample is sent; therefore five weeks is about the usual time which has slipped away *since the typhoid germs were received by the patient into his body from the water supply,* before the laboratory man receives a sample from it! Now, *two* weeks is probably the usual maximum for typhoid germs to live in water, even if the water be stagnant and in a dark place. When it is heaving, changing, exposed to the sun and wind and current, or flowing fast, as in a river, the life of disease germs in it is even shorter, and the chances of their dispersion and disappearance by the mere physical losing of themselves are almost infinite. To apply laboratory methods to finding typhoid germs in the ordinary sample of water taken from the suspected supply five weeks after the cases were infected, would be like shooting at the place where a flock of ducks *had been five weeks before.* " Hunting for a needle in a haystack " is discouraging enough in itself, but suppose you *knew* the needle had been carefully removed before you began your hunt!

The laboratory man who examines water does so, not in the hope of finding typhoid germs,— he does not even try to look for them, as a rule,— but to find certain other signs of excretory pollution. Curiously enough, these signs are often of more real value to Public Health than would be the finding of the typhoid germs themselves, were that practicable; but to explain how this is, would be out of place here. The point is this:

The laboratory tests of the supposed routes of infection in any given case are made by methods and for ends wholly different from those which the public fondly imagines. The results obtained are often far more valuable than the public realizes or expects. At the same time, the definiteness of these results, because of the facts already outlined, are far inferior to those obtained by the laboratory examination of infected persons — in brief, the information obtained by the laboratory from the examination of "samples" usually requires elucidation and explanation in the light of all sorts of other information, sociological, meteorological, topographical, geological, etc. Considered thus, the laboratory work is nearly invaluable, but, taken by itself, almost as nearly worthless.

The happy ignorance displayed by those who think that an analysis of water, or milk, or food, even the most thorough, can in itself and by itself give useful sanitary information is equalled only by the joyful confidence of the southern darkey in a rabbit's foot.[2]

The true position of the laboratory in the co-ordination of public health workers which will rule in future organization, has been achieved but seldom.

[2] The British Medical Association at its annual meeting, held 1912, passed the following resolution: "That this con-joint meeting of the sections of State Medicine and Bacteriology unanimously desires strongly to urge that no opinion as to the quality of a water for dietetic purposes should be arrived at on bacteriological evidence without a local and topographical inspection of the sources of the supply made by a competent observer."

The Public Health laboratory man of to-day has ceased to be the leader in public health endeavor which he once was, partly because he has been swamped with routine work in the lines he has himself developed, but chiefly because, being a laboratory man, the very nature of his work has kept him indoors, out of and apart from the stirring fields of human life in being. Perfect enough in his own technic, he has perforce lost touch with all but his own work, and other lines of public health, more closely involved with the outer world, have passed ahead of his.

The laboratory man of the future will get out into the actual daily lives of the people and communities he serves. He will know outside conditions as well as those in the laboratory. He will work more closely with the engineer and the epidemiologist. He has his own place which they can fill no more than he can fill theirs, but he must understand their work, and they his, much better than at present.

Moreover, the engineer and the epidemiologist suffer from the present disassociation of the laboratory quite as much as does the laboratory man himself. Field work moves lamely, oftentimes, from lack of laboratory knowledge, just as laboratory work is oftentimes inert from lack of field knowledge. During the last few years the frequent transfer of laboratory men into the field work of epidemiology and engineering has evolved a set of men who recognize this fully. But it is not by

COMMUNITY DEFENSE 131

transferring laboratory men to other fields that the laboratory can be developed. It is by putting the laboratory itself into the field — and only so — that this can be accomplished.

In field work, and in research, so much neglected of late, the laboratory man will find his future, and he will not deal solely, as at present, with infectious diseases. True, the venereal diseases must be added to the present list of those for which routine laboratory facilities are provided. But some non-infectious diseases may become preventable diseases, if their causes are discovered, and the Public Health laboratory of the future, acting in conjunction with the physiologist and the pathologist, may find therein usefulnesses now undreamed of. Finally, as we slowly learn the true personal hygiene of food, clothing, sleep, exercise, etc., the Public Health laboratory will take its share in the greatest, but least developed, of all Public Health procedures, namely, the physical advancement of the race.

SUMMARY

The Public Health laboratory finds its chief functions to-day in the detection of infectious persons (sources), and in the identification of infected things (routes), as means to the end of abolishing those sources and blocking those routes. The average public health laboratory has been swamped with routine, cribbed, cabined, and confined until useful research has almost died out and real knowledge of outside conditions has been lost. The engineer and the epidemiologist have progressed fast and far by active contact with the needs of the outside world, and the laboratory can attain its proper future only by like development.

CHAPTER XII

COMMUNITY DEFENSE

THE PUBLIC HEALTH STATISTICIAN

IN the development of the new public health principles, the laboratory came first. It dealt with the *causes* of disease at first hand, as well as with their *sources* and their *routes* of transmission. On laboratory findings all modern public health is based, although in practice the laboratory is necessarily limited, for daily service, to those diseases the causes of which are known.

But in its earlier work, the laboratory, inheriting somewhat the environmental teachings of the older school, paid more attention to *routes* than it did to *sources,* especially to the routes constituted by (a) water and (b) general surroundings. This focused attention on (a) sanitary engineering and (b) disinfection. It was in the earlier laboratory period that the sanitary engineer and the disinfector developed highly. It is true that the engineer deals almost solely as yet with but one *route,* water; and that therefore his efforts necessarily relate almost solely to the intestinal infections, mainly to typhoid fever. Nevertheless, so valuable were his services in reducing this disease, that engineering work was hailed at one time as the solution of all public health questions. Now the epidemiologist leads the van, because he deals not with *some routes,* of *some* infectious diseases, but with *all sources* of *all* infectious diseases.

STATISTICS AS THEY WILL BE

But, through the work of the laboratory man, the engineer, and the epidemiologist, has for long been heard a still, small voice, offering a framework to bind them all together — to give coherence, correlation, and proportion — to outline the future, as well as to record the past, and, above all, to direct the present. This was the voice of the vital statistician. Much abused, laughed at, neglected, he is, or will be, guide, map-maker, intelligence department, all in one; he is, or will be, like the cost-of-production scientific manager of modern business, " the most indispensable man on the staff."

True, his professional ancestors were helpless old gentlemen, raising their feeble voices in very feeble chants. A dry-as-dust historian of the wars of ancient Greece could lend more aid to a modern football team than the old-time statistician furnished to public health endeavors. Even now the new vital statistician is scarcely yet full-born. Hardly a health department now in existence collects in full or uses to full advantage one-tenth the information that it really needs. (A notable exception should be recorded here, the Richmond (Va.) Health Department under E. C. Levy.) The laboratory man has made some good statistics in his own field; so has the sanitary engineer — sometimes, alas, not wisely, but too well; the epidemiologist, also, from sheer necessity: but the new vital statistician has only begun to move. When he does move, fully equipped, alert, he will systematize, organize, and *use* the rich data so far largely wasted, this very life-blood of public health endeavor, accurate, complete information concerning the way humanity reacts to human ills. Internal public health organization has been like the old-time factory, full of good workmen, but each working only his own line, with no one person knowing much about the business as a whole. At the end of the year the business, drifting along, perhaps showed a doubtful profit, perhaps a loss, but so long as bills and wages were somehow paid, who cared? Public health requires exactly the kind of man who has changed the face of business in the last fifteen years, a man who understands all parts of it, but does none himself; a man who knows costs in each department in proportion to production, and where to cut cost, increase production, save time, unnecessary work, and waste in general; alas, in health departments, a man to stop the one-half, now done uselessly in wholly wrong directions and to force development of the other half, now much neglected or left undone completely.

It is the vital statistician who must do this: collect the facts and set them forth inexorably, with mathematical precision. When it is done, our health departments will no longer use up $30,000 for garbage, with the probability that not a single life will be saved thereby, while spending $12,000 on *all other* health department efforts combined. Nor will a health department spend for terminal disinfection one-tenth its annual appropriation, to save no lives at all,[1] while using but one-fiftieth its appropriation for tuberculosis, which kills five times as many people as all the diseases usually "disinfected" put together.

It will be said: "You are confusing vital statistics with health department finance; vital statistics deal with deaths, not money." Exactly — and that is just exactly what is wrong with them. Vital statistics are now, in short, not *vital;* they deal with Death, not Life, with the "finished product" only of our slack, slipshod methods. They ought to deal, not merely with dead bodies, but who they, living, were, and why and how they died, and above all with why they were not saved. Suppose the factory manager knew at the end of the year merely his total product! Suppose that even this piece of information related, not to the way business went last year, but to the way it went *five years before.* "Historical records, and mighty poor at that," a modern public health man said in bitter scorn of the statistics of a neighboring State. The modern scientific manager must know not merely the total product, though he must know that, and to the minute, not to five years

[1] In tuberculosis, where terminal disinfection would be valuable it is not often done.— *J. A. P. H. A.*, April, 1913, p. 311, M. N. Baker.

before; he must know also all about the product, the kind, the quality, the cost, and why it is not better for the price. The modern vital statistician must know not only deaths, but why the health department is not stopping them; what its funds are; how they are spent or wasted; what work is being done; how much of value each division does; and all to the one end of saving life, not to the end of stopping nuisances, removing garbage, or cleaning streets — all admirable ends no doubt, but not life-saving ends.

But, it will be said, "Very well, but you are wrong in stating that Vital Statistics deal with Deaths. They deal with more than Deaths — they deal with Births and Marriages and contagious diseases also." "Yes, nominally; but to what useful end for public health?" [2]

"Birth records quite often affect inheritance of estates in later years." True, and very useful to the inheritor they are when the time comes, but what has that got to do with *saving life* now? Marriage records also are invaluable in their own way, but they do not reduce tuberculosis one-tenth of a tenth per cent. Contagious disease reports, then? Surely they are important? Yes, but not as they are, too often, now collected. Misleading information is sometimes worse than none at all.

[2] Birth records, if they led to immediate investigation to see that the child was cared for properly, would be true public health data.

STATISTICS AS THEY ARE

The best way to show what public health vital statistics as they are to-day mean, or do not mean, is to give the story, true to life, as any one who knows will quickly see, of the very basis of such statistics, the actual facts as they occur amongst the people.

Mrs. Anybody says to Mr. Ditto: "I am afraid Tommy has scarlet fever; I think he must have caught it when he was in the city." "Call Dr. A." "Yes, but they say he will report it, if it is scarlet fever. I'm nearly wild now with work. When the children are at school all day I manage somehow; with you and the children quarantined at home for a month I should go insane. I'll call Dr. B.; they say he never reports anything. I'll tell the neighbors it is scarlet rash. That's not a lie. It's a rash, and it certainly is scarlet. I'll let the children go to school, but I'll keep every one away from Tommy. I'd hate to think any other child got it from our children, but I guess that will be all right. Tommy is not very sick. Don't go telling any one he is sick. I'll tell the children not to, either. We don't want to have the milkman or the grocer afraid to call."

So Mrs. Anybody plans, and so it is carried out. But her heart is bigger than her head, and her plans go strangely awry.

She puts Tommy in a room by himself and runs over to a neighbor's for an egg or a cup of flour. When she

COMMUNITY DEFENSE

comes back the other children are lined up in Tommy's room, solemnly inspecting the rash he proudly demonstrates to them. Next morning Tommy is "real sick," and after breakfast the mother puts up the other children's school lunches alternately with running in to Tommy's room to give him water or to hold the basin while he vomits or just to kiss and soothe him.

Poor, loving, hard-working mother! She has done this same through all the ages, this taking of infected discharges from the sick child, on her hands, to be put later in the other children's food. No, she won't kiss them good-bye; she has been kissing Tommy; that is, she won't kiss any but the smallest one, who looks nearest to crying. She wipes that one's mouth with her apron before she kisses it — *she does not wipe her own!* Not that wiping either matters, for Tommy's mouth discharges are already in the lunch the little one marches out with, under its arm.

About 10 A. M., the empty house and the wailing child get on the mother's nerves. So she calls in a neighbor. " Tommy's sick. I want to go to the store to telephone the doctor. It's only scarlet rash. I won't be gone more than a minute, but I'm afraid he'll get out of bed or something. Will you keep an eye on him?"

The neighbor comes in, the baby on her arm, for is it not scarlet rash? But prudence strikes her suddenly, and she sets the baby on the floor before she peeks in at Tommy. "Hullo!" "Hullo, Mrs. Neighbor!" a feeble little voice replies. She steps in further, leaving the door open to keep an eye on baby. "Well, Tommy, how do you feel?" "Not very well," and he begins to vomit. She snatches a basin, holds his head, and in a moment surrenders him to his mother, and then takes her baby hurriedly home. A speck of vomit-spray has hit her hand. She did not notice it. The baby's fingers rest on it a moment, before it is dry; a minute later the baby sucks that finger. At home she sets the baby down and, conscience-smitten, changes her dress (*she does not wash her hands!*) and thereafter feels all right again because she thinks that *now* she can't give it to any one, even if it is scarlet fever; besides, the doctor said it was scarlet rash.

Meantime, Mr. Anybody, summoned by his wife, hurries home in terror, finds Tommy still quite alive, growls, fusses, brings in some wood, pumps a little water, and then steps into Tommy's room, "just inside the door for a minute," before going down-town again. Tommy, with feverish, flushed face and heavy eyes under his tousled hair, calls feebly, "My daddy, my daddy"; and, of course, Mr. Anybody steps to his bedside to pat his head and kiss him, before hurrying back to business.

That night Tommy is worse; sorrow is on the family in earnest. Next morning Tommy is much better; the prayers and tears of the night before are forgotten; the mother, weary but joyful, lets the other children in to see him; "just for a minute now, but, anyway, he is so much better," and they all race out to school, shouting and laughing.

About five days later, Susan, the youngest, is not feeling very well towards evening, vomits during the night, is delirious next morning, with sore throat, swollen neck, and rash; and Dr. B. comes again. Serious measures are taken. The other children, in tears, are spirited away to a cousin's house to stay lest they should get it, and because the mother can't stand the strain of nursing the sick and caring for the well also.

Tommy has had it mildly, and by this time is up and about, wandering disconsolately through the empty house. To all inquirers the mother bravely maintains that Susan has only the scarlet rash and tells them Tommy will go back to school in a day or two. "I just sent the other children away because they were so noisy," she explains guiltily, wishing very earnestly that it was really so.

Next day Susan is *better*. (I am writing this — and therefore I make it thus. In real life, poor little Susan often dies, instead.) Every one is cheerful again. Tommy is sent, very unobtrusively, to school because "he mopes at home, without a soul to play with." He is beginning to peel, and, in a day or two, is in much demand amongst his schoolmates, presenting them with souvenirs of flakes of skin they treasure as curiosities. Not that these scales do harm, despite the old beliefs. It is not the peeling, which everybody sees, that does the mischief, but the unnoticed slightly red sore throat that Tommy carries with him, and from which he infects his hands (and every one he touches) and shoots out infection in his mouth-spray as he chants his lesson, or whispers across the aisle, or sings in class.

And so the old, old story works itself out inexorably. One of the other children, staying at the cousin's, develops a slight sore throat. Were there an epidemiologist at hand, posted on the history of the child, to scan the enlarged papillæ of the tongue, note the large glands, and see the filmy membrane on the tonsils, the case would be recognized as scarlet fever, *sine eruptione,* i.e., without a rash. But as it is "it's only a sore throat." No physician sees her, because the cousin argues thus: "If it were my child, I'd have in Dr. A., but Mrs. Anybody wouldn't thank me for running up another bill here, unless the child is really ill; she's having Dr. B. now, for Susan, twice a day. I'll wait a day or two, anyway."

The sore throat heals, and the cousin feels she made a good judgment. But meantime the sore-throat girl has been sleeping with the cousin's little girl, and she develops it, too, but it also passes off. Then a week later, the cousin's little girl's school-chum, in a different school from Tommy's, has scarlet fever proper. Dr. A. attends, and reports it. The Health Department puts a placard up; the children are kept out of school; the father is kept at home; the whole population turns its eyes on that family and wonders where they got it. The village wiseacres, over the village bar, remind each other of the slough behind the house, or that the garbage from the family was never removed all summer. They say the well is shallow, " nothing but surface water," or the house is damp, or too much shut-in by trees, or any other fatuous foolishness that enters their empty heads. The mayor gives out a statement to " allay popular excitement." He brands as malicious all statements that scarlet fever is rampant. There is but one " sporadic case," originating no one knows how. It is carefully quarantined, and " the Health Department believes the outbreak is well in hand and practically stamped out." The Women's Club demands the fumigation of the schools; and the epidemiologist, if only he were present, would gaze reflectively at Tommy's slightly red throat, and gnash his teeth, and swear.[3] Poor Dr. A. who only did his duty, is blamed for all the trouble; and Dr. B. keeps mum. When, presently, Dr. C. is called to one of Tommy's schoolmates, he hesitates. He has not seen much scarlet fever, and he thinks, " perhaps it *is* scarlet rash — whatever that may be." He attends the child two or three days, and then he begins to ponder whether or not he had best put the responsibility on the Board of Health; so at last he calls up Dr. D., the Health Officer. But Dr. D. has troubles of his own. " Do you say it is scarlet fever ? "

[3] *Editor's Note.*— We regret the epidemiologist should do this, but we propose to give the facts, no matter whom they hit. Besides, we do not blame the epidemiologist much under the circumstances.

"Well, I don't know. I want you to go and see." The H. O. is perplexed. He does not want the reputation of finding a second case, after the Mayor has stated that there is only one; so he tells Dr. C.: "If you report it, I'll placard the house, but I don't want you to report it, if you are not sure." At this Dr. C. waits a day or two more, but finally reports it. Meantime a week of association of the other children with the sick one has elapsed, because Dr. C. did not *quite* know the finer points in recognizing mild scarlet fever early.

By this time, between the unconscious activities of Tommy and Susan, who are back at school, well oiled by Dr. B.'s advice, to keep the scales from showing, and of Susan's sister and the cousin's little girl (none of them recognized officially as scarlet fever), some twenty or thirty children in the two schools have been infected. Some of the pupils have had scarlet fever before and so escape this time. In others the disease is mild and passes unnoticed. In others "scarlet rash" develops. But several develop frank scarlet fever, not to be denied even by Dr. B. who, to give him credit, has begun "to get a little scared," and so reports one or two well-marked cases to relieve his conscience. Two or three deaths occur, and then the schools are closed, but not the Sunday schools, or churches, or private sociables, or moving pictures, and so it drifts.

Now, see how all this affects vital statistics. The Health Department, in its annual statement, gives as the first case that school chum of the cousin's little girl.

We know that there were four cases before that — Tommy and Susan, and Susan's sister, and the cousin's little girl — but these do not go down upon the books at all. The Health Department adds thirteen more cases; that is, all those cases attended by Dr. A., faithful, conscientious man; about half of Dr. B.'s cases, those he had after he "got scared"; and some of Dr. C.'s, but only those he was absolutely certain of, not knowing scarlet fever very well. Dr. D. had no cases, because, being health officer, the mothers felt that he would *have* to report them, and so did not call him.

The fact is, that any epidemiologist would find that there were forty cases, but the books show fourteen.

Then consider the deaths. Two were reported properly as due to scarlet fever. But one of Dr. B.'s, really scarlet fever, not quarantined while ill, is reported "acute Bright's disease," because the doctor dare not say it died of scarlet fever after treating it a month without reporting it. It is quite true the child had Bright's disease, but it had Bright's disease because it had scarlet fever. Another dies of meningitis, due to middle-ear infection, the result of scarlet fever, but being meningitis, this death also goes in a different column. The more or less spoiled ears and the more or less spoiled kidneys of twenty other children who recovered never are recorded on the books at all.

Hence, fourteen cases where there should be forty; and two deaths, where there were really four, are recorded officially as scarlet fever.

This instance exemplifies practically the whole situation; mild, unrecognized, and concealed cases; cases to which physicians are not called at all; mistaken diagnoses; a superficial report covering a few of the severer cases only; death reports correct so far as they go, but not showing the relation of the death to the preceding disease. This occurs, not occasionally, in a few communities, with scarlet fever only, but, almost every time, in almost every community, with almost every one of the infectious diseases.

The returns from Anybodyville are small in number, it is true; but multiply these by all the similar communities which make similar returns. Anybodyville reports two deaths and fourteen cases from scarlet fever, where there were four deaths and forty cases. This is "only" two deaths and twenty-six cases wrong. But if one thousand communities report similarly, our statistics are wrong two thousand deaths and twenty-six thousand cases.

Moreover, see how the percentages are twisted and tangled. Two deaths from fourteen cases is about 14 per cent. Two deaths from forty cases is 5 per cent. Four deaths from fourteen cases is 28 per cent. Four deaths from forty cases is 10 per cent. When we remember that the number of cases of scarlet fever, and of other diseases, is often calculated from the deaths by the percentage which the deaths *usually* are of the cases, we find that we can calculate the cases from one hundred deaths of scarlet fever (on the above returns) as seven hundred, two thousand, three hundred and fifty, or one thousand — how *very* valuable!

SUMMARY

The vital statistician of the future will be the scientific manager of a business department, for, through the epidemiologist working in the field, he will know where the diseases *are,* not where they *were,* and he will know which disease demands the most attention. He will know also what resources, in men and money, the health department has, with which to fight its battles. The correlation of these two factors has seldom been achieved, although in life insurance it has long been known that their inter-relations were the absolute *sine qua non* of success. Any business man's first step in reorganizing public health for actual service would necessarily be (a) to determine what requires to be done; (b) to determine what there is to do it with. The maximum *required* returns from the minimum *necessary* expenditure should be the only motto. To secure this information, no one but a statistician knowing statistics, but knowing men and things as well as figures, can succeed. To confine his work to deaths, even to cases, from preventable diseases, is to study output only, with no regard to income. To study income, as is so widely done, without regard to whether that income is spent to achieve lessening of disease and death, or merely for nuisances or smoke inspection, is simple madness.

CHAPTER XIII

ADMINISTRATION

The administrator of public health is confronted as we all are in every line of life by the necessity for discriminating Æsthetics or what we would like to have, Hygienics or what we need, and Economics or what we can actually secure.

Too often the administrator, tempted by the desire to please, or yielding to the pressure of demands made by the unknowing, or even himself suffering from confusion of mind as to the relations of cause and effect in public health work, has devoted his department to such æsthetics as might be within his grasp, neglecting entirely or largely the truly hygienic measures he might have undertaken. Quite generally, out of date laws, ordinances devised by the most ignorant of lawmakers, have compelled the most wise administrator to subordinate measures he knew to be valuable to those he knew to be useless for the suppression of disease and death. Thus it comes about that many health departments are loaded down with expenditures in money, men and time, for non-health purposes which, good in themselves, or at least harmless, absorb the forces which might be devoted to directly improving health or to preventing dis-

ADMINISTRATION

ease. There are those who say, "If the object is a good one, why object to the Health Department doing it? — does it matter to the citizen whether or not the garbage is removed by the Health Department or the Street Department so long as it is removed?" This argument would be passable, if all health departments had unlimited money and were manned by experts in every line of municipal care. Then there would be no administrative objection to handing over, not garbage only but charities and corrections and the customs collection, inland revenue and conduct of the schools to health departments. As it is, however, with inadequate means for even their proper functions, and with experts trained in medical lines or cognate subjects, the health department supervising utilities of this kind is a splendid example of carefully constructing a razor, and then needlessly using it as an axe.

But there is a much deeper and more serious error in such division of health department work, *the* great error in recent public health administration, the error of educating the public, not by words, but deeds, to the conception that æsthetics, the miscellaneous methods of municipal housekeeping, the cleanliness of externals, the neatness and promptness of the garbage and ash collections, are the essential weapons against disease. As well say that the ordinary order and cleanliness of the wellkept home creates it a fit hospital for contagious diseases.

Many a health department now standing high in the

estimation of the citizens and gaining praise in all directions from those who see its spectacular operations for cleanliness, smoke prevention, etc., is really not only a total failure in suppressing disease (except sometimes in suppressing the fact of its existence) but is actually misleading the public and building up false ideals which ultimately damage the community and the race, causing loss of life and money immensely in excess of the comfort or economy secured by such municipal cleanliness. Municipal cleanliness is excellent in itself — it is the substitution of municipal cleanliness for the real disease prevention that we deplore.

The ideal health department of to-day organized to suppress disease and death, not to clean streets or to fuss about the plumbing, need at the present time consist of but five or six technical divisions corresponding with the basic essentials, man and his surroundings. These are the Epidemiological Division, dealing directly with the individual, sick or well; primarily for the discovery of the infected persons, secondarily for the control and elimination of the sociological conditions contributing to infection.

For the surroundings of man is needed a Sanitary Engineering Division dealing with all the essentials of construction and operation of public or private utilities which bear upon the promotion of health or the prevention of disease and death, i.e., for the control of the physical sources and elimination of the physical routes of transfer of disease.

ADMINISTRATION

For the bookkeeping of this combination an alert active Vital Statistics Division is essential — not for the bookkeeping of dollars and cents but of human lives and health.

A Laboratory Division is required, to apply to the activities of the epidemiologist and the sanitary engineer the most advanced of chemical and bacteriological work. This division should be, like the others, fully equipped in men and money for every known form of investigation into the preventable diseases, and the analysis of anything which may be useful to the prevention of disease, especially for the analysis of sewage, water, milk and other foods, drugs, poisons, etc., in brief, for the analysis of man and of those surroundings of man which affect him disastrously, or favorably.

A figure now new in health department activities should be a permanent feature in the future, although at the present time the work he could do would be largely investigative and advisory, i.e., a trained Physiologist, devoting himself to the study of physiology as it relates to hygiene, i.e., to the attainment of physical perfection and efficiency, with comfort; and the maintaining of the same through a long life. The division which he heads should be equipped for every form of investigation into food values, labor conditions, especially in factories and in schools (the universal factories which all must enter) and should devote itself wholly to studies developing ultimately to the place where actual legal enforcement of valuable regulations relating to hygienic conditions may be made, not limited to mere physical surroundings but also including hours of labor, housing and many other problems now largely drifting.

In those communities where medical school inspection is under boards of health this physiological division might well directly control it. When under well equipped school boards the actual operations of the medical inspection may well be conducted in close cooperation with this division.

Of the non-technical divisions a most important one is that which engages itself with Publicity. Although usually best managed as a subdivision of the administrative mechanism, this division should be regarded as equally important with any other and should be in the closest touch with all of them, keeping records of and publishing promptly the work of each department in an acceptable form; explaining the principles and aims of the whole in each of the operations it undertakes; and posting the public on the actual conditions found, the problems they present, the remedies proposed and the results of remedial operations. This division might well use lectures and similar methods as well as newspapers and its great keynote should be — must be — the truth, the whole truth, and nothing but the truth.

The Administrative Division should itself be the center of the whole mechanism, seeing with the eyes and ears of all the other divisions, planning, correlating, directing, demanding returns for all monies spent and shifting the weight of a large General Fund from division to division as the needs vary. The finance subdivision should be equipped with expert accountants who are well posted on the needs as well as the mere outgo of each division. Administration is a business as well as an art in any large operation, whatever its purpose. But in public health work it is a business and an art which is supposed to be and therefore should be, energized and directed to the general physical welfare of mankind; enlightened with a fine appreciation of relative values; and guided by the great general's discrimination between the essential and the non-essential, the things that win as distinguished from the things that merely seem to; the things that threaten in appearance only, as distinguished from the apparently innocent things that really mean great mischief.

The head of the administration should be unhampered by any Board of Strategy. The chiefs of his own divisions, picked properly to begin with, should form his best council, and he should seldom need other. Political exigencies should control him no more than they control the military officer in the face of the enemy. The Board of Health of to-day is often a mere anachronism, built up when there were no experts, with the hope that, all being blind, combining one with another would manufacture sight between them. Now that men really versed in public health can be secured, nothing is gained by placing a merely official board in actual control, **for if** composed, as many boards may now be, of experts, they tend to take the place of a single executive; while if composed, as they usually are in practice, of inexpert laymen, or worse, physicians inexpert in public health, but who are nevertheless under the supposed halo of a medical degree, they do more harm than good. A very level-headed board of very just, farseeing, men will sometimes be found whose advice in conference is of real value to the administrative head [1] but these are the exception, and many Boards are merely excuses for political control and diversion to spectacular ends of monies which should be expended on the objects for which they were appropriated, i.e., for public health and the diminution of disease and death. Such an ideal Health Department, in close touch with every agency dealing with social or physical improvement, will be in close touch with the medical profession. It should not be burdened with general hospital management nor as a rule with the management even of a contagious disease hospital: but it should control the situation completely so far as such agencies have to do with the spread or prevention of spread of all infections. In the hospitals as in the schools and factories its rule in this respect, should be quite absolute. The Administrative Division needs a law subdivision and usually a police subdivision also. The reporting of contagious diseases by physicians should be enforced, but with a properly conducted Epidemiological division, it should

[1] It has been the writer's good fortune to work under such Boards in both Minnesota and London.

ADMINISTRATION

be rather the rule for the Health Department to discover and report cases to the Medical profession for treatment than that the medical profession should report infection to the Health Department. Indeed until the existing status is reversed, until Health Departments know more of the whereabouts of infectious persons than the whole medical profession can tell them, the abolition of infections will remain a dream of the future.

We have spent many years blaming the medical profession for laxity in reporting, without stopping to think that if every medical man reported correctly every infection that he sees however trivial, still infection would be continued through those cases that call no physician, and through infected persons who are not sick. Until Health Departments do more — much more — than perfunctorily placard only reported cases, there is no inducement to physicians to report their cases; and until Health Departments are equipped with means and insight to provide properly in all respects for the infected persons thus cut off from their usual associations and operations, such segregation is an injustice that the public will continue to resent.

So long as governments permit infection to go unchecked, relying footlessly on physicians' reports alone, the persons who unwittingly become infected should have rights in suits of damages against such governments. This has been the enlightened ruling with regard to typhoid fever contracted from a public water supply. There is no reason why it should not be extended to every form of infection however contracted.

SUMMARY

The Health Department of the future will be a business department for the suppression of disease and death and the promotion of general high health, not as at present a pseudo-charitable institution for the conduct of a jumble of activities, a muddle of municipal cleansing and æsthetics.

The administrative head will be an expert, not a political exigency; and his lieutenants will be men of training as deep and broad as his own, each in their specialties. These will be epidemiology, vital statistics, sanitary engineering, bacteriology and chemistry: each organized on the broadest basis for actual efficient accomplishment of the ends of public health. The administrative division, well equipped for financial supervision and executive direction of the whole, will nevertheless be devoted to the one end of accomplishing results; and will include as an important feature a publicity bureau or division; while as the next development of the future, a trained physiologist to study the questions of hygienics as applied to the community may well be added.

The sanitary inspections, back yard cleanings, street sweepings, smoke preventions, weed cuttings, removal of dead animals, garbage disposals and other like physical functions of a municipality will be relegated to the

ADMINISTRATION

Public Works or Street Departments, relieving the Health department of physical burdens and setting them free for their true sociological work with human beings.

This scheme is not by any means for big cities only. The smaller cities and towns and rural districts must be combined into populations of 20,000; or even less in sparsely settled areas. For each of these a similar department should exist. The present reproach that half the population, i.e., that half residing in the country, is practically without public health agencies, must be removed and every citizen treated equally wherever he lives. This is not mere abstract justice but also a real need.

The realization that infection moves back and forth from urban to rural districts and vice versa should give to all the clearest understanding that disease in one depends upon disease existing in the other as much as in itself and neither city nor country can free itself alone but both must act together. The summer colonies of city people in the country, the constant visits of country people to the cities, the growing interchange in every way, have done away forever with distinctions from the public health standpoint. No government that fails to recognize this can succeed in public health campaigns.

CHAPTER XIV

COMMUNITY DEFENSE APPLIED

TUBERCULOSIS IN GENERAL

PREVIOUS chapters have outlined the general principles which govern modern public health efforts. The present chapter will show the specific applications of these principles to one specific infectious disease, namely, tuberculosis. This disease is selected because the same principles that apply to all other infectious diseases apply to it and because it is the most important of all the diseases now recognized as really *preventable,* with the exception of the venereal diseases.

Tuberculosis, in all forms, is due to the growth, somewhere in the body, of a certain germ, exactly as diphtheria and typhoid are due to the growth, in the body, of certain germs. There are many very definite individual differences, in the size, shape, manner of growth, etc., of the three different germs of these three different diseases, and these differences make it perfectly possible to distinguish each germ from the others, just as any farmer can distinguish oats, corn, and potatoes from each other.

But just as there are different varieties of potatoes,

COMMUNITY DEFENSE APPLIED 159

so there are at least two varieties of tuberculosis germs which affect human beings. One variety is what is known as the human tuberculosis germ proper. The other is found chiefly in cattle and is therefore called the cattle tuberculosis germ (the bovine tuberculosis germ), and this name is given to this variety even when it is found in the human, as it sometimes is.

HUMAN TUBERCULOSIS

One of the most important differences that the germs of human tuberculosis, of diphtheria, and of typhoid fever show amongst themselves is not a difference in size, shape, etc., but in the parts of the body each selects. Thus the diphtheria germ flourishes chiefly in the nose and throat; the typhoid germ flourishes chiefly in the intestine and perhaps in the blood; while the human tuberculosis germ will flourish almost anywhere in the body, glands, bones, joints, intestine, kidney, brain, lungs. This selection is no mere accident, although we do not know how it comes about. All three germs enter the body chiefly by the mouth, conveyed thereto chiefly by the *hands,* but also more or less through food and milk, and, in the case of typhoid fever, through water and flies. On entering the mouth, all three germs, which are of course far too small to taste or feel, are swallowed in the food, milk, etc., in which they happen to be present, or merely in the saliva, if, as is most usual, they reach the mouth directly or indirectly from the fingers. Once swallowed, all three pass into the stomach, where many are killed by the acid there present, the survivors, if any, passing on into the intestine. On this journey from mouth to intestine, some are left, of course, by the wayside, stranded on the tonsils, throat, gullet, etc. Here at once is shown their respective peculiarities. Of all the diphtheria germs that are thus swallowed, practically only those that are stranded in the throat will flourish; those diphtheria germs which pass on into the stomach or intestine are destroyed or pass out harmlessly. On the other hand, typhoid germs, if stranded on the throat, do not flourish there, nor do those which reach the stomach flourish in that organ. It is only those typhoid germs which survive the journey until the intestine is entered that can succeed in producing typhoid fever. The human tuberculosis germ has a still longer road to go. Not only must it pass mouth, stomach, and intestine; also it must be absorbed from the intestine into the blood, as the food is; but it does not grow in the blood. The blood is only a river, by which it can be carried to a favorable developing ground. We do not know at all why human tuberculosis germs, entering the blood thus, should finally settle and grow in a joint in one person, in a lung in another, in a kidney or a gland or a bone in another. However, this is the way in which these different forms of human tuberculosis develop. The old idea that human tuberculosis of the lung (consumption) is contracted chiefly by breathing the germs directly into the lungs has been definitely upset. The lungs are infected from the

COMMUNITY DEFENSE APPLIED 161

blood-stream chiefly, just as are the other internal organs, bones, and joints.

Another and, from the public health standpoint, an even more important difference exists. Diphtheria germs developing in the throat, and typhoid fever germs developing in the intestine, can readily escape from the body; in the case of diphtheria, through the mouth and nose discharges; in the case of typhoid fever through the bowel, and sometimes the bladder, discharges. It is the escape by these channels of these germs from the body which makes these diseases "catching" or "infectious" or "communicable," for if they could not escape from the body they could not reach other persons and therefore could not be "catching." But in human tuberculosis, most of the places where it develops,—bones, glands, joints, etc.,— are not connected with any opening of the body by which the germs may leave the body. These forms of tuberculosis have no great highway to the outside lying at their doors to carry the germs out to other persons. Practically only in human tuberculosis of the lungs is such a highway provided for the human tuberculosis germs, although sometimes in bladder, kidney, and intestinal tuberculosis. But in the latter forms, the germs do not, as a rule, pass out by the highways provided for them in such condition or such numbers as to be of serious importance in propagating the disease. In human lung tuberculosis, on the other hand, the windpipe, throat, and mouth form a highway, along which the germs may escape from the affected lung in such enormous numbers that twenty-four billion per day have been detected in the discharges (sputum) from the lung of a single advanced case, although the average number from the average case is usually " only " four or five billion daily.

Thus it comes about that human tuberculosis of the lungs is the only common form of human tuberculosis which is much to be feared as infectious. Practically all the chief forms of human tuberculosis are derived from the sputum of cases of human lung tuberculosis, carried chiefly by mouth-spray and on the hands, and if cases of human lung tuberculosis did not act to spread infection to other persons, all forms of human tuberculosis would quickly disappear.

Moreover, even human lung tuberculosis is not infectious in the early stages, i.e., when the germs are growing in the lung tissue, but have not yet reached the air-passages; because, until then, the germs cannot escape into the windpipe and so by the throat to the mouth. When in the later stages the germs reach the air-passages the way for the escape of the germs to the outside and so to other mouths is " open." Persons in this stage of tuberculosis are called " open " cases, and it is therefore only the " open " cases that are seriously to be feared as infectious. Because of this, tuberculosis is not spread much in the public schools. Many school children are tuberculous; but open cases are not common. Sometimes the former should be taken out of school for their own good, but the latter alone are dangerous.

THE ABOLITION OF CATTLE TUBERCULOSIS FROM THE HUMAN

Although the cattle tuberculosis germ differs from the human tuberculosis germ somewhat in size, shape, etc., the most important public health difference is this: the cattle tuberculosis germ seldom produces lung tuberculosis in the human. It produces bone, gland, joint, etc., tuberculosis, but lung tuberculosis hardly ever. Consider how important this fact is. It means that *cattle tuberculosis existing in a human can very seldom be conveyed from that human to another human.* It other words, cattle tuberculosis may be transmitted from cattle to man, but practically is not further transmitted from man to man. To prevent cattle tuberculosis in the human, we do not need to take into account existing cases of cattle tuberculosis in the human, but only existing cases of cattle tuberculosis in cattle. If we free our cattle of cattle tuberculosis, we shall free our humans of cattle tuberculosis also; and this is the only practical way that cattle tuberculosis in the human can be abolished unless and until the human race abandons the use of *raw* cow's milk.

THE ABOLITION OF HUMAN TUBERCULOSIS

How can we abolish human tuberculosis? Exactly as we can, and some day shall, abolish any and all other infectious diseases, by killing off the germ that causes it; exactly as we have almost abolished the race of buffalo by killing off the existing buffalo. We know well enough that when the last buffalo is dead, no man, however wise, no government, however powerful, could ever produce another buffalo. So, once the existing diphtheria or scarlet fever or tuberculosis germs are all dead, there is no way under heaven by which these particular germs could be produced again. Those which exist now are not "evolved from dirt" any more than are buffalo or roses. Those which are living to-day are simply the descendants of those which existed yesterday and so on, just as in the case of buffalo or roses, back to the dawn of history. Once any race of plant or animal is wiped out, it can never be redeveloped; and the tuberculosis germ, just as well as the germs of diphtheria or typhoid fever, can be abolished exactly as the megatherium or dinosaur has been abolished, i.e., by killing off the existing individuals.

"But consider the enormous numbers and the tiny size of germs and that they are present *everywhere,*—in air, water, food, milk, dust; in and on everything we touch or taste or handle. It is quite impossible to kill them all."

True, *germs* are everywhere but *not disease germs*. We know some fifteen hundred or more species of germs and hardly fifty of these produce disease, while only two, already mentioned, produce tuberculosis in the human. That these germs are very small and cannot be slaughtered individually like buffalo, is true, but it

COMMUNITY DEFENSE APPLIED 165

is also true that their very minuteness means that billions can be slaughtered at a time, if they are only kept together. As to tuberculosis germs being everywhere, all over, outdoors and indoors — this is *not* true. No more important fact in public health has ever been formulated than this, due to that keen leader in public health, Chapin of Providence: *The germs that produce disease* are *not* ubiquitous, *not* in dust everywhere, water everywhere, milk everywhere. They are chiefly, almost wholly, *in the bodies* of a relatively few people, or animals; and when they escape from those bodies, where alone they find the peculiar food, high temperature, abundant moisture, and darkness which they need, they promptly die or become harmless. Even in water, milk, food, etc., into which they may be introduced from infected persons, their lives are short, and they must quickly reach a new living victim, or die.

To abolish any one race of disease germs is far easier than to destroy some much larger things. Thus to abolish flies means not only killing all flies, indoors in all houses everywhere, in all stables everywhere, in and around all dwellings everywhere, but also throughout all fields and forests, mountains and valleys everywhere, because flies are hardy outdoor beings as well as indoor beings. They can breed and flourish almost anywhere, where any kind of food, even in vanishing quantity, is to be had. Moreover, they can move of their own volition with promptness and despatch, have quick eyes and quicker wings to escape designing enemies, and in a thousand ways can take care of themselves.

Disease germs, in contrast with the fly, are very tiny and helpless particles of protoplasm, having no eyes to see an enemy, no nose to smell him, no means of running away from him. They cannot flourish on almost any food, but need the living tissues of the human body; they cannot grow at almost any temperature, but must have the heat of the human body. In brief, they are not merely indoor plants; they are incubator plants and·cannot grow, thrive, or reproduce themselves in nature, except in the incubators, which our bodies (or, in a few cases, animal bodies), provide for them. Hence if we were able to take a visual census of all the living tuberculosis or scarlet fever or diphtheria germs in the world we should see them, not in the dust everywhere, the water everywhere, the food everywhere, etc., but in a very few places only, and those places would be, in almost all cases, the bodies of humans (or animals).

Indeed, we can foretell just about what the census of tuberculosis germs in any district of the temperate zone would show. It would show about one person in every five hundred of the population carrying a large number of active, living, growing germs in the lungs,— germs that were escaping to the outside and reaching other persons' mouths. It would also show a number of other persons in whom the germs were present in joints, bones, glands, etc., but not escaping to others; and it would

COMMUNITY DEFENSE APPLIED 167

show a number of persons affected in the lungs, and later likely to develop to the point where the germs could escape, but practically harmless to others so far. Beyond this, hunt high, hunt low, search garbage barrels, manure heaps, dead animals, dusty streets, sewage, water, foods, milk, etc., and human tuberculosis germs, alive, growing, capable of producing the disease, *would seldom be found.* True, in the immediate neighborhood of the " open " cases, the sputum they throw out, their mouth-spray, and their hands, would show the germs; and things they spit into, mouth-spray into, or touch, would show for a short time a few; but these would be dying or already dead, holding out danger to other persons only during the short time which elapses between leaving their happy homes in the human lung and death outside from drying and starvation. This applies, not to tuberculosis germs alone, but practically to all the germs of the ordinary infectious diseases, anthrax and tetanus forming two chief exceptions, both comparatively rare diseases in civil life.

No person energetic enough to advocate the abolition of the fly should hesitate a moment to advocate the far simpler, smaller, easier, and far more important work of abolishing those germs that alone can make the fly a danger.

In brief, the method, and, I believe, the only rapid, complete, effectual method of abolishing human tuberculosis, is this: find the " open " cases and prevent the spread from them of the germs they alone throw out in numbers and condition to be feared. That means, find the one person in every five hundred whose infection threatens all the rest, and supervise him just enough to keep his discharges from entering other people's mouths.

How is this one person in every five hundred to be found? Not without hunting, not without ingenious, skillful, deliberate, sagacious, well-trained hunters, epidemiologists as devoted and persistent in their work as the average insurance agent is in his,— men who devote themselves to the abolition of tuberculosis as wholeheartedly as any merchant does to making money.

And how? Where shall we begin? Must we canvass the whole population one by one? True, that would do it, but epidemiology has found a simpler, keener, more scientific, far more economic plan, illustrated for typhoid fever in a previous chapter. Begin with the known cases and search the zones of infection surrounding each for mild, unrecognized, and concealed cases. (In tuberculosis the search for carriers is probably unnecessary, certainly at the present time.)

"But why not concentrate on the incipient lung case, the case that may be cured, and by preventing this case from going on to the 'open' infectious stage get rid of danger to others thus, instead of by attention to the open case?"

For several reasons the abolition of tuberculosis through care of incipient lung cases only cannot at present be accomplished.

1st. Because incipient cases, in the truly incipient

COMMUNITY DEFENSE APPLIED

"non-open" stage, are discovered, perhaps are discoverable, in a very small percentage only of their total number.

2nd. Because a large proportion of the true incipients so found would *not* go on *in any case,* whether found or not, to the open stage; and the time and money and efforts spent in finding and supervising them would have been relatively wasted.

3rd. Because a certain proportion of the incipients so found *would* go on, *in any case,* to the open stage, and thus become infectious cases, despite all efforts. In these alone would the efforts expended be of service in preventing new cases. The trouble is that, in the truly incipient stage, it could not be determined whether or not the case would so develop.

4th. Because the time and attention devoted to incipients, in the effort to prevent them becoming open cases, would imply, as it has, too often, so far implied, neglect of the advanced "open" cases, from which the danger of infection is so immensely greater.

5th. Because if all the truly incipient cases were discovered they would form a mass of persons so great as to be beyond handling properly by any at present even dreamed of force of attendants, etc. If, as at present, only a very small proportion were found the actual situation would not be materially changed.

"Would you then cease the care of incipient cases in sanatoria, and concentrate wholly on sanatoria or hospitals for the advanced case?"

No. First, because the tuberculosis sanatoria for incipients, intended though they are for incipient cases, really handle very many "open" cases, and to that extent prevent new infections; secondly, because the tuberculosis sanatoria for incipients do, in a measure, fulfill their proper function of cure for incipients and even early "open" cases to some extent and hence save life. But as a means of *abolishing* tuberculosis, the ordinary tuberculosis sanatorium for incipient cases is quite hopeless.

The thing to do first is, find the recognized "open" cases, whether they be in early, advanced, or late stages, and place *them* where *they* can spread the disease no further.[1] Then search the "zones of infection" surrounding them, i.e., their relatives and associates, for mild, unrecognized or concealed cases, and also for incipients, handling all "open" infectious cases thus found in the same manner. This system would begin at the right end by *stopping further infection,* and would incidentally find those early "open" and "non-open" incipient cases wherein sanatorium treatment would be of most avail.

SUMMARY

Human Tuberculosis is a typical infectious disease, and it must be handled on the same principles as any

[1] The County Sanatoria of Minnesota, Wisconsin and many other States furnish exactly this place. They spell the abolition of tuberculosis if properly developed.

COMMUNITY DEFENSE APPLIED 171

other infectious disease; hence, by blocking the routes of infection, but chiefly by finding the *sources* and preventing spread thence.

Of the five great routes of infection,— water, food, flies, milk, and contact,— human tuberculosis travels chiefly by contact, through sputum, mouth-spray, and hands, directly, or almost directly, from patient to prospective patient. Practically, it is spread exactly as scarlet fever or diphtheria is spread.

Public flies and public food supplies are comparatively insignificant conveyors of this disease. Public water supplies are almost negligible, and public milk supplies act chiefly in conveying cattle tuberculosis to man, although, if the milk be handled by tuberculous humans, it may convey human tuberculosis also.

It is evident, then, that blocking the routes of human tuberculosis, since the chief one is contact, really involves the far more important measure of finding the sources, just as in scarlet fever, or diphtheria. If these sources are found and prevented from gaining access to the routes, the routes may be disregarded. The measures for finding the human sources, practically the "open" cases of *lung* tuberculosis in the human, are epidemiological and have already been discussed in principle before (Chapter V).

The transmission of cattle tuberculosis from cattle to human contrasts with the transmission of human tuberculosis from human to human in that it occurs almost wholly by one definite route, raw milk; scarcely, if at all, through contact.

Since this one route can be absolutely, easily, promptly, and inexpensively, blocked by the simple process of pasteurizing or otherwise killing the germs in the milk, there is no reason why we should await the equally absolute, but more difficult, much slower, and very much more expensive abolition of the sources, i.e., the elimination of tuberculous cattle from all herds, although the latter should be gradually pushed to completion for economic reasons, whether the use of raw milk be abandoned or not. The measures necessary for finding the animal sources (infected milch cows) are the well-known tuberculin test of herds, with proper repetitions, and the elimination of the tuberculous animals.

Serious enough as cattle tuberculosis in the human is, its prevalence, nevertheless, is much less than that of human tuberculosis, its infectiveness from human to human is nearly negligible and the pasteurization of milk would eliminate it from the human. Hence, if our efforts were concentrated wholly on abolishing human tuberculosis from the human, more cases and more deaths would be prevented in one year's work, than efforts directed to abolishing bovine tuberculosis from cattle, however successful, could possibly achieve in many years.

CHAPTER XV

THE CONTROL OF DIPHTHERIA, SCARLET FEVER AND MEASLES

WITHOUT attempting to describe the technical details, a sketch of the modern procedures, such as should be clear to all laymen dealing with the schools, is worth while as an illustration of the advances and advantages of the new practice.

In past times, and of course even now, an outbreak of diphtheria in a school was considered the signal for " immediate action "— so far, so good.

But that action often consisted chiefly in the closing of the school for disinfection, and reopening it again as soon as this ceremony of purification was performed. Should the scare be great enough the school, perhaps, all the schools of the community, were closed for weeks, to prevent spread of the disease amongst the children. The length of the period of closing was pure guess work. The time at which the schools were reopened seems usually to have been decided by the condition of " scare " in the community. The outbreak sometimes ended in correlation with some one or more of these varieties of action. But very often, the outbreak spread while the schools were closed, and if not, took a new lease of life when they were reopened. The children, excluded from nearly all schools, were not effectively forbidden to meet at play or work outside the school.

The panic-origin of the method, its lack of clean-cut object, its "hit-or-missness," rendered it wholly unsatisfactory as a scientific means of controlling the disease, to say nothing of the upset and loss of school time, the disturbance of the school finances, the degeneration of the school children thus forced to an uncertain vacation, not provided for at home.

The new method never interrupts the school at all. It brings to bear only so much pressure as is actually needed. The principle is simple — remove the infection from the school. The practice is equally simple — discover by cultures of the children's throats [1] those who may be infected; send them and their brothers and sisters home, and continue all the school operations as before with the remaining children.

The infected children who are sent home must be followed to their homes and prevented from conveying their germs to uninfected companions out of school. They are in fact isolated until such time as (a) the germs they carry are shown by proper tests to be nonvirulent or (b) the germs disappear, of themselves (as very often happens) or under treatment (lemon-juice or kaolin).

[1] Not forgetting the throats of the teachers and of the janitor, also. Often cultures from noses also are advisable.

DIPHTHERIA AND SCARLET FEVER 175

In institutions, a further step may be taken. Through the Schick test, the children who are immune to diphtheria, ranging perhaps an average of 50 to 60 per cent. of all the children, may be kept together and all infected children may freely associate with them, without danger of disease. The non-immunes are likewise kept in another group, and watched by culture and clinical observation for the development of further cases. This group may receive antitoxin also.

The advantages of this simple procedure are too obvious for need of expression here.

In scarlet fever, a very similar procedure was introduced and developed to a high degree of perfection by A. J. Chesley in Minnesota.

The principle is exactly similar, but since the, as yet, hypothetical scarlet fever germ cannot of course be recognized as is the diphtheria germ, clinical observation necessarily takes the place of cultures.

As in diphtheria, the children are examined at the school; but by direct inspection of the face, tongue, throat, glands, chest, sometimes one foot: those showing signs of recent or developing scarlet fever are sent home, with their brothers and sisters, and the remaining children continue at school safely.

Because scarlet fever may be incubating in children for several days before giving outward signs, the procedure is further modified from that used in diphtheria to the extent that the inspection just described is repeated every day for a week. All children still without signs of scarlet fever may then continue at school as safely as may those who, in a diphtheria epidemic, have had eliminated from amongst them the diphtheria infected throats.

In scarlet fever, exactly as in diphtheria, the following up to their homes and isolation there of the infected children is an essential to prevent spread from them amongst school children after school hours, or amongst non-school children they may otherwise encounter.

Quite similar methods may be and have been successfully applied to measles. In this disease, the infectious period begins three or four days before the rash, with the beginning of the earliest symptoms, which usually are first observed as, and often taken to be, those of a heavy cold, with reddened eyes and hoarseness. All schools should stand ready to eliminate from amongst their pupils *all* sick children — for the sake of the child itself, but even more for the sake of its associates. Such children should not only be sent home, but should not be returned to school again without a medical inspection, preferably by a school physician.

SUMMARY

Some day infection will be so well controlled outside the schools that infected children will not enter schools; and then, school outbreaks will be unknown. But in the transition period from the diluted barbarism of today to the conditions just outlined, diphtheria, scarlet

DIPHTHERIA AND SCARLET FEVER 177

fever and measles can be detected and eliminated from schools, and best by keeping the schools open, not by closing them, provided the methods outlined above are followed.

Not only do these methods keep the schools free of infection and hence make them "the safest place in town," but also the follow-up system, also outlined, provides for the elimination of out-of-school infection from the community.

Of course, both within and outside the schools, the epidemiologist, thoroughly posted on the natural history of the diseases he deals with and keen to trace its sources and its routes, is a *sine qua non*.

CHAPTER XVI

VENEREAL DISEASES

We know how to prevent any infectious disease the moment we know where its sources are, if we can control them.

In tuberculosis we are getting control slowly of the two main sources and routes, tuberculous cattle and the raw milk from them for bovine tuberculosis, the human consumptive and his mouth discharges for human tuberculosis.

In typhoid fever, scarlet fever, diphtheria, etc., exactly the same things are true and exactly the same sort of principles are to be applied, and have been applied most brilliantly and successfully.

In the venereal diseases, however, although the same principles of course remain as true as ever, their application to the sociological conditions of the day have yet to be worked out upon a practical footing.

The people, as a whole, have overlooked the fact that more than half of the cases are innocently contracted, and attach a stigma to all that is deserved by few. Hence one great difficulty in the discovery of cases, and *the* difficulty in dealing with them after their discovery.

VENEREAL DISEASES 179

Moral suasion has been tried for thousands of years, and venereal diseases have increased instead of diminishing.

The elimination of these diseases from the race is the practical duty of the professional public health man and he every year considers it more seriously.

Preliminary steps have been taken to determine the extent of the problem, with appalling results, but these should rather urge to more immediate and strenuous action than result in inertia and despair.

It has been pointed out elsewhere that education of the average person to avoid other diseases is, while worth while, of little final value, because infection cannot be recognized by laymen, nor can the channels by which it travels be so continuously blocked in ordinary life as to avoid unrecognized infection; hence that it is the duty of the community to eliminate infection from itself entirely and free its members of all need for personal defence. This is everywhere recognized as sound governmental policy in relation to other dangers, fire, thieves, invaders — why not in relation to these more constant, more inevitable and more insidious foes?

The sources of infection are the venereally infected persons who now exist. Unfortunately these are not confined to any group or class or profession, but are scattered everywhere.

The routes of transmission are intimate contact, but not necessarily sexual, or when sexual, not necessarily guilty; yet of a nature making the tracing of **transmis-**

sion rather a delicate task. The control of the infected heretofore has not been recognized as anything like so important as the control of scarlet fever or diphtheria infection, despite the far greater damage that they do.

While prophylactic disinfection may be and has been practised with great success in naval and military circles, the apparent endorsement that arrangements to this end give to illicit relations makes it difficult to enjoin or even urge them in civil life.

Hence the venereal problem, while gradually taking shape, is as yet hardly concrete enough to permit formulation of a definite program.

All that can really be held as absolutely demonstrated is this: however the solution may be reached, it necessarily must involve one, two or more of the simple principles established for the control of other infections: immunization, avoidance of the sources, blocking of the routes, elimination of the sources; the latter being the highest ideal. The first is as yet hypothetical; the second has totally failed to eliminate these diseases from the race, although a perfect method when practicable and practised. The third is the only method successful to date on any scale large enough to offer evidence of its efficiency. The fourth is as yet a dream.

Education of children in sexual hygiene cannot but be of benefit in some cases and while no final solution of the problem, paves the way to it by doing away with the false modesty that envelopes these great scourges

VENEREAL DISEASES

of the race in a sanctified mystery of misery that conduces greatly to their successful propagation.

Wherever "hush" is heard, wherever mystery and mysticism reign, there we find superstitious practices and suffering beyond belief.

"The dark places of the earth are full of cruelty"— and doubtless after all is said and done, publicity will prove if not the solution, the first step to the solution, of this our greatest present day public health question.

CHAPTER XVII

THE CONCLUSION OF THE WHOLE MATTER

THE DOING OF IT

IF previous chapters have succeeded in the very earnest attempt they made to show what the new public health principles are and how they have become established, the one momentous matter in public health still left unsolved is this — why, why, why are not these principles observed? If we know how to do it, why is it not done?

Chiefly, because the general public does *not* know. They still believe religiously the theories that were beginning to be discarded in scientific circles twenty years ago. To any one who has discussed these subjects before lay audiences it becomes most evident that people the most refined and educated still believe, concerning public health, almost the same things that the most ignorant hold.

How many people believe that gold wedding rings rubbed on the eye will cure styes? That green apples cause colic? That ear-rings improve sight? That a copper wire round the waist prevents rheumatism?

CONCLUSION OF WHOLE MATTER 183

That horse-hairs soaked in water become snakes? That only nasty medicines cure? That whiskey is good for pretty nearly any ailment? That the moon affects lunatics? That tuberculosis is hereditary? That measles is inevitable? That typhoid comes from dead weeds in drinking water? That red flannel (must be *red!*) is good for sore throats? That sewer gas is poison? That smallpox can be telephoned from one person to another? That mosquitoes come from decomposing leaves? That malaria is due to night-air? That robust people do not have smallpox? That scarlet fever scales are infectious? That raw beef-steak is good for a black eye? That drinking cow's blood cures consumption? That the smell from a horse stable cures consumption? That if medicine is good for sick people, it must be still better for well ones? That eating turnips makes one brave? That onions cure or prevent smallpox? That dead bodies necessarily breed a pestilence? That rusty nails produce tetanus (lock-jaw)? That goats in a stable save the horses from glanders? That in epidemics schools should be closed? That Cuban Itch is not smallpox? That washing the exterior of the body removes disease from the interior of the body? That children *ought* to have " children's diseases "? That the younger they have them the better? That all colds are due to cold? That fever is due to heat? That brain-fever comes from excitement or strain? That people " gradually run down, and it turns into " typhoid or tuberculosis? That backache indicates kidney trouble? That vaccination is worse than smallpox? That you "mustn't give in to" disease, but fight it off by force of sticking at your work? That cold weather is healthy because it kills germs? That oxygen kills disease germs? That small flies grow into big ones? That cancers have roots like a tree; roots which can be drawn out with the cancer, if care is exercised? That grapeseeds produce appendicitis? That cherrystones swallowed may grow a cherry tree in your stomach? That pickles sour the milk of a nursing mother? That a meat diet tends to produce a quarrelsome disposition? That there is no danger of infection from a sick child unless a doctor has pronounced exactly what the particular disease is? That mild attacks of infectious diseases are less infectious than severe ones?

So long as this jumble of pure myth, current tradition, childhood misunderstandings carried over unconsciously into the serious repertoire of adult conceptions, control and form the basis of procedure for the public health thought and action of the race, so long will public health be what it largely is to-day, a farce and laughing stock.

Until these absurdities are definitely combated and eliminated, the teaching of the truth is retarded, for the public tend, not to replace the superstition by the fact, but to adjust one to the other, making a more hideous jumble than ever. Curiously also, it is the fact that is modified in such adjustment, not the superstition. We, as a race, pride ourselves on our cold-blooded, calculat-

CONCLUSION OF WHOLE MATTER

ing analysis of things, our elimination of old-world formulas, of old-world rules. Yet in public health, nothing is too ridiculous or far-fetched to find ready believers — eager strivers after mystery, people who prefer complicated non-sequitors to simple facts.

Four of the most common fallacies the writer's experience of public discussion has elicited are illustrated here, and the reader may easily test his own state of knowledge by asking himself what answers he would give to the questions here presented:

THE CHIEF OBJECTIONS

1. If the disease germs are not evolved afresh from dirt or decomposition, but are descendants of their forefathers, where did the first disease germ come from?

We do not know. Where did the first wheat come from? Or the first horse? We know that we can get no wheat *now*, except from wheat, nor horses except from horses. These germs are plants or animals, exactly as wheat or horses are. That they are tiny no more changes this law of descent than does the enormous size of a whale or of a redwood tree make them exceptions. "All life from life" holds true in nature through the whole scale, from germ to human beings. Besides, under the microscope, we *see* the germs "descending" from their forefathers.

2. If dirt does not breed disease, then why are dirty people so subject to disease?

Dirty people are no more subject to disease than

clean. Infection, if it reaches either, may yield disease, in either; if it reaches neither, neither will suffer. If an infectious disease enters a household, the dirtiest people will not spread it, despite their dirty habits, *if they avoid the one specific " dirt "* (the discharges of the patient) which alone is harmful; the cleanest people will not fail to catch it if, in their general cleanliness, they neglect that same specific " dirt." True, dirt, carelessness and disorder offer some indication whether or not the people who show these characteristics would have the sense, or take the trouble, to avoid the one dangerous " dirt," should it appear. On the other hand, cleanliness, thrift, and system indicate characters likely to handle infectious " dirt " with the same care they show in other matters. But the dirtiest people who make the proper efforts to avoid infection can and do many times escape, remaining as dirty as they please in other ways. The cleanest people who neglect or do not know the methods can and do suffer.

3. If you tell people " dirt " does not breed disease, you are praising dirt — upsetting all the careful uplift all the best people have attempted for many, many years.

Suppose a *water*-pipe is leaking in your house, flooding the floors and damaging everything. Suppose that when the plumber is hurried to the rescue, he tests the *gas*-pipes, finds a leak, stops it, and tells you all is well. What would you say? True, the *gas* leaked; it was right to stop it; but the *water* goes flowing on! Sup-

CONCLUSION OF WHOLE MATTER 187

pose to your objections he replies: "But think how bad the effect would be on our campaign against gas-leaks, if we failed to urge that gas-leaks must be stopped, whether that stops the water-leaks or not. If I admit that gas-leaks have no connection with water-leaks, you would let the gas flow on. I *must* make you believe the water-leak depends on the gas-leak, else you won't fix the gas-leak." Stopping gas-leaks cannot help water-leaks nor vice versa. Reducing disease will not make people "clean," nor will making people "clean" reduce disease; only the one "cleanliness" of avoiding infected discharges will gain this end.

4. Why do you talk so much about disease? Teach healthy living, keep the body strong, well clothed, well fed, and you need not fear disease, especially infectious disease, at all.

This is a fallacy so widespread that even physicians teach it, in good faith, without considering that they themselves would never let their own children, be they never so healthy, run with a measles case, or mumps, or scarlet fever, unless their children had had the disease before. If the teaching is not good enough for practical application to physician's children, it is not good enough for public health.

You see, every one knows that children who have had measles very seldom take it a second time, and this without regard to whether they are robust or sickly, healthy or weak. Every one knows, too, that children, healthy or sickly, who have not yet had measles, almost invariably catch it if they are exposed. Practically, the same is true of scarlet fever, mumps, whooping cough, smallpox, chickenpox, etc. It is not so true of tuberculosis, diphtheria, or typhoid, since those who have had tuberculosis, diphtheria, or typhoid may take it again; although again without regard to whether they are healthy or sickly.

In measles and the other diseases like it, persons exposed who do not contract the disease, escape, not from good health, but just because they have within their bodies a certain antidote to the particular poison of that particular disease. Any one can prove this to himself, if he will think a moment. If general good health really did protect against these diseases, a child who could not catch measles, *because protected by his general good health,* could not catch scarlet fever, either, for the same general health would save him from them both. But every one knows that the child who cannot catch measles (because he has had it) must nevertheless be guarded from scarlet fever, unless he has had that too. In brief, an attack of these diseases gives, in most persons, an immunity; that is, an antidote is formed, which then protects them from having it again. But there is a *different antidote* for each disease. Having had measles once is excellent protection against measles, but it is no protection at all against scarlet fever or mumps or any other illness.

In diphtheria an antidote is formed, but often disappears again, and therefore this disease may be suffered

CONCLUSION OF WHOLE MATTER

more than once. In typhoid also an antidote is formed lasting a year or two. We know something, and are learning more, of this antidote against typhoid. We do not know yet much about that which perhaps protects against tuberculosis.

Now, no one dreams that the antidote for measles can be developed by diet, exercise, or clothing; by fresh air, drugs, or anything in fact, except by suffering an attack from the measles germ. Nor can any one seriously believe that the antidotes for typhoid or chickenpox, etc. (except that for smallpox vaccination takes the place of an attack of smallpox), can be developed except by equivalent means. If "good health" will not protect against any of these diseases, taken *one by one,* how can "good health" protect against *all* of them taken together?

So we might deal with fallacy after fallacy, all based, however, on two.

POPULAR FALLACIES

The first of these is that infectious diseases come from "general bad surroundings." The truth is that they come solely from certain germs growing in the body, and practically the only sort of "bad surroundings" which causes infection is association with one of these infected bodies or with its discharges.

The second great basic fallacy is this, that "general good health" protects against infection. The truth is, that the only true protections against germs we know are, first and best, to keep them out of the body; and, second, to have within the body the *special* antidote for each *particular* germ. We vaccinate against smallpox, but that does not save us from typhoid fever. We vaccinate against typhoid fever, but that does not save us from smallpox. If we could vaccinate against every disease (as perhaps some day we shall be able to do) we would be safe, despite the germs, at least while the protection lasted, and after that we could vaccinate again.

But how much better to abolish the germs, which means guarding all persons in whom they are; and then we would never need any sort of vaccination!

Surely, the thing to do for one's own sake, and still more for the sake of our associates, is to find the infected persons, or animals, that alone can cause disease in the true sense, and keep them so protected while the danger lasts that they will do no harm. Then, when their stock of germs is dead and done with, remove all the restrictions.

NEW FASHIONED QUARANTINE

You will say that that is only old-fashioned quarantine. It is, in principle, but modern practice changes it so completely that, practically speaking, new-fashioned quarantine differs from old as much as motor cars differ from camels, although both are means of locomotion. In the first place, old-fashioned quarantine did not pick out *all dangerous persons,* but took the sick who

CONCLUSION OF WHOLE MATTER

form but *part* of the infected, and also took the well who were found with the sick, including thus some who were not infected, and kept all these practically in prison, in their homes, or ships, or wherever else they were staying. Thus, not alone were many infected persons overlooked and many uninfected persons wrongly held, but also the disease spread oftentimes from those infected who were in the net to the uninfected who were kept in with them, so that old-fashioned quarantine, while it protected the community but partially, meant often poverty, disease, and death to those caught in its toils. No wonder the very name of quarantine makes many people shudder.

New-fashioned quarantine is not a blanket method, blunderingly catching in its blindfold grip both sick and well, the harmless and the harmful, indiscriminately. New-fashioned quarantine requires definite detailed knowledge applied with care and patience, not mere force.

Now, every one wishes infectious persons handled so that infection ceases. The infectious persons themselves do not wish to spread their own infection. The thing that chafes and riles the average person is not restriction but unjust restriction; either restriction of non-dangerous persons, or restriction of some of the dangerous only, while others just as dangerous go free.

No mother minds the exclusion of her infectious child from public school, if her neighbor's infectious child is excluded also. Every physician would report his cases if every other physician did so too.

Here then is the solution, based on human nature, on common sense, and on the most scientific knowledge. Find, through the methods of epidemiology, of the laboratory, and of the vital statistician, skilfully combined by experts, these dangerous persons, whether sick or well — these only dangerous persons, those who carry on them or in them, germs of infectious diseases. Set all others free, but keep these persons, not in old-fashioned quarantine, but under such control that their discharges will not pass to others; and do not measure the length of that control by fixed time limits, blind and unjust as quarantine itself, but measure it wholly by the length of time the germs remain in or on the body. The moment that the germs have left those persons they are no longer harmful and they should be freed.

To do this properly means intimate attention and supervision of infectious persons by men who know their business and do nothing else. If one such man to every 20,000 persons began, to-morrow, everywhere, his work, infectious diseases in ten years would have vanished and would have become mere history.

SUMMARY

This, then, is the conclusion. The old ideas have passed; the new are no longer theories but facts; the methods they require are not untried; they have been practiced for years in many places. The details are

CONCLUSION OF WHOLE MATTER

worked out, the field is ready, the scope and cost are known. All that remains is to apply the methods already developed to all infections, thus wiping them all out, once and for all. The way is clear, what remains is to follow it; the method is known, what remains is to carry it out; the thing we, as a race, for centuries have prayed for, can be done; all that remains is to do it.

Each generation of Americans pays now for infectious disease ten billion dollars at the least, *and has the diseases, too!* Why not pay one-tenth this sum and rid ourselves of all of them forever?

APPENDIX I

ISSUED BY THE INSTITUTE OF PUBLIC HEALTH
(See Over)

These Diseases are Reportable by HOUSEHOLDERS, under penalty; and by PHYSICIANS who know or suspect their presence, under penalty.

	I. Immediate Report Required	II. Terminal Disinfection by M.O.H.	III. Isolation of Patient	IV. Placard Required	V. Quarantine of Associates	VI. Quarantine period of those exposed (dating from last exposure).
Smallpox (1) (2)	+	+	+	+	+	14 days
Scarlet Fever (1) (2)	+	+	+	+	+	10 days
Diphtheria (1) (2)	+	+	+	+	+	12 days
Measles (1) (2)	+	+	+	+	+	16 days
Poliomyelitis (1) (2)	+	+	+	+	+	
Cerebro-spinal m-n-g-t-s (1) (2)	+	+	+	+	+	
Typhoid (1) (2)	+	+	+			
Chickenpox (1) (2)	+	+	+			14 days
Whooping Cough (2)	+	+	+			14 days
Mumps (1)	+	+				18 days
Tuberculosis (1)	+	+				
Rabies (1)	+					
German Measles (1)	+					16 days

NOTE.—(1) By the Provincial Health Act.
(2) By Provincial Regulations.
(3) Leprosy, Bubonic Plague, Asiatic Cholera, Erysipelas, Glanders (in human), and Anthrax (in human) are also reportable, under penalty, by householders and by physicians.

APPENDIX II

ISSUED BY THE INSTITUTE OF PUBLIC HEALTH
(See Over)

These Diseases are Reportable by HOUSEHOLDERS, under penalty; and by PHYSICIANS who know or suspect their presence, under penalty.

	VII. Return of Patient to School permitted only after	VIII. Private Funeral	IX. Incubation Period	X. Prodromal Period
Smallpox (1) (2)	Scabs gone	+	12-14 days	3-4 days
Scarlet Fever (1) (2)	If Desquamation, albumen, throat, etc. O. K. 6 weeks from rash		2-6 days	1 day
Diphtheria (1) (2)	3 weeks or 2 negative cultures	+	1-3 days	½ day
Measles (1) (2)	If Desquamation, cough, etc., has ceased, 3 weeks from rash		9-11 days	3-4 days
Poliomyelitis (1) (2)		+	Unknown	3-4 days
Cerebro-spinal m-n-g-t-s (1) (2)		+	Unknown	
Typhoid (1) (2)	8 weeks from first symptoms		5-23 days	7 days
Chickenpox (1) (2)	Scabs gone		15-17 days	½ day
Whooping Cough (2)	6 weeks from first whoop		7-14 days	7 days
Mumps (1)	4 weeks from enlargement		14-25 days	1-2 days
Tuberculosis (1)			3-12 mos.	
Rabies (1)			3 wks-3 mos.	
German Measles (1)	3 weeks from eruption		14-16 days	½ day

NOTE.—(1) By the Provincial Health Act.
(2) By Provincial Regulations.
(3) Leprosy, Bubonic Plague, Asiatic Cholera, Erysipelas, Glanders (in human), and Anthrax (in human) are also reportable, under penalty, by householders and by physicians.

APPENDIX II

SYLLABUS OF PUBLIC HEALTH TEACHING

As an example of the sort of material which should be presented to school children, the following syllabus already in use in Minnesota is appended. This was prepared by the writer in co-operation with Mr. C. G. Schulz, State Superintendent of Education. It was intended to supply to the public school teachers of the State a condensed but accurate outline which they should then put into their own words for the information of their pupils. Syllabus No. 1 might well be taught in all grades; syllabus No. 2, in whole or in part, in all grades; syllabus No. 3, in the sixth and higher grades; while syllabus No. 4 is applicable rather to the eighth and higher grades, thus including the high and normal schools.

Elementary and simple as the information given may appear to those who are conversant with all phases of Public Health, the writer's experience is that the most enlightened and well-educated of those of the laity who received their education in times past, when nothing of this nature was offered, find in these leaflets a very great deal of information which is to them new, intensely interesting, and often quite revolutionary. These leaflets have been prepared with the utmost care and submitted to a number of the highest authorities in each subject treated of, in order to assure the strict accuracy and up-to-dateness of the statements made.

Prepared by H. W. HILL, M.B., M.D., D.P.H.

No. 1. GERMS AND DISEASE

1. Not less than 1500 kinds of germs exist — but only about 50 to 75 produce disease. Remember these two classes: (a) disease germs and (b) all other kinds.

2. Germs of all kinds are simply tiny plants (or animals); some spherical, some more or less sausage shaped; so small that from 100,000,000 to 200,000,000 might lie side by side on a thumbnail, yet could not be seen.

3. Germs of any kind never "evolve" from dirt. They, like other plants (or animals), come only from predecessors. They increase in number by single germs separating into two; then each of these grows and likewise separates; this is repeated about every twenty minutes, when conditions are good for the germs, giving about 1,000,000,000 descendants in ten hours.

4. Conditions good for the germs mean: (a) much water, (b) the right food, (c) the right temperature, (d) darkness, (e) the right atmosphere. These differ for different kinds of germs; most disease germs find the living body the best place for them: when they leave it, sunlight and drying soon kill or disable them.

5. Many different kinds of germs that do not produce disease flourish on or in our skins, noses, mouths and intestines all the time.

6. We all pass our germs on to other people whom we meet,

APPENDIX 199

and they pass theirs on to us. But this does no harm, unless disease germs are present too. Disease germs are found chiefly in persons who have or have had some infectious disease.

7. Neither disease germs nor other kinds can jump or fly from one person to another; they are *carried*, chiefly in the discharges from the nose, mouth, bladder and bowel.

8. These discharges are exchanged chiefly by mouthspray, sputum, and hands; also by things touched by mouthspray, sputum or hands.

9. Mouthspray means the small, sometimes invisible, drops of liquid from the mouth that we throw out when we sneeze or cough or talk or sing or shout; in quiet breathing they are not thrown out.

10. Sputum is spit — the liquid from the mouth, generally mixed with liquid from the nose or lungs. When it is thrown out where it can be stepped on it may be carried to other people, chiefly on feet of animals or shoes of humans.

11. Hands, most of all, carry all kinds of germs from one person to another because hands carry mouthspray, sputum, nose, bladder and bowel discharges to other people's hands, and to things that other people touch.

12. Although most healthy people's germs are not disease germs and are therefore harmless to other people, it is hard to tell when even healthy people may get disease germs from some one else — therefore

13. Try to keep your *hands* out of your mouth and nose, and away from other discharges, unless they are washed well before (for your sake) and then washed well afterwards (for others' sake).

14. Try not to handle any food, cups, spoons, or other things which other people may put into their mouths, unless your hands are first washed clean from your own nose, mouth, bowel and bladder discharges.

15. Try not to leave any fresh moist discharges from your body where other people or animals will touch them, or step on them; or where flies will get at them and carry them to other people's food.

16. Water and milk, as well as food and flies, carry discharges to other people. Therefore don't let your discharges get into or on any of them.

17. Try to get other people to be as careful as you are.

18. *Try not to let other people pass on their germs to you,* ESPECIALLY IF THEY HAVE ANY KIND OF DISEASE GERMS (tuberculosis, typhoid, scarlet fever, measles, etc.).

No. 2. FOOD AND WATER

1. Food and water, next to ourselves, are the most important physical things, for they are what *we* are made of; we are about 70 per cent. water, the rest food.

2. When first born, we weigh about 7 to 8 lbs., as adults 120 to 200 lbs. The difference comes from *part* of the food and water we have taken in.

3. A large part of the food we eat does not become part of us, but is burned up as fuel to keep our bodies going. Children usually gain weight fast; because they eat more than they burn up. Adults usually do not gain weight much; because they burn up about as much as they eat.

4. Our food comes, directly or indirectly, from the soil — the crust of the earth. Therefore we are made of the crust of the earth. So are all plants and animals.

5. The crust of the earth is made up of about 80 elements — about one-fourth of these go to form our bodies. These include carbon (found in diamonds and coal), oxygen, hydrogen (found in air and water), nitrogen (found in air), phosphorus, sulphur, sodium, potassium, calcium, magnesium, iron, chlorine, iodine, fluorine, etc. (found in various salts in food and water).

APPENDIX

6. We cannot feed ourselves on these elements; they must be combined from the soil, air, and water by bacteria and plants into forms we can use; often we get the combinations we need by eating animals, which themselves live on plants.

7. The chief combinations we can use are known as fats, carbohydrates, proteins, vitamins, salts, water.

8. Fats (including oils) are found in fat of animals (lard, suet, etc.); and oil of plants (olive oil, peanut butter, etc.). They consist of carbon, oxygen and hydrogen.

9. Carbohydrates are combinations of carbon, oxygen and hydrogen also, but differ from fats in the way they are put together. They include starches and sugars.

10. Proteins form the main substance of white of egg, lean meat, lean fish; and are found also in plants. Proteins are combinations of carbon, oxygen, hydrogen, and *nitrogen*, with phosphorus, sulphur, and other elements present in various amounts.

11. Vitamins are peculiar things, essential to nutrition; they are present in raw plants, fresh milk, etc.

12. Salts are combinations of calcium, magnesium, etc., with oxygen, hydrogen, etc.: they are useful in many ways in the body; calcium especially in forming bone.

13. Water is the great solvent and carrier of material from place to place in the body: blood is nearly all water, and carries food and oxygen to the muscles, brain, etc., and waste matter from them to the kidneys and lungs.

14. Since the really living parts of us are largely protein, only protein can be used to repair waste or add to our bodies. We cannot long survive on a diet without protein in it.

15. But part of the protein we eat and all of the fat, oil, starch and sugar is useful only as fuel.

16. All of this fuel is burned in the body, in the muscles, brain, etc. Our lungs make the draft for the fire, and let out the "smoke," carbonic acid. (See "Air," par. 4 and 5.)

17. Fats and carbohydrates, if not burned up at once, are stored as fat; some carbohydrate is stored as animal starch (glycogen) in liver and muscle. Sugar and starch in excess make people stout.

18. Fat in the body is stored fuel, ready for use on occasion. Very thin people have no reserve fuel, very fat people have too much.

19. Children under one year should have water and human milk — nothing else, if possible.

20. Children over one year should be carefully taught to use all good "adult" foods; fats, carbohydrates, proteins, vitamins, salts, water.

21. All growing children need protein, to *add* to their bodies as well as to repair waste. Sugar, starch, and fats, are good fuels for children.

22. Healthy adults need protein for repair of waste only.

23. Boys from 9–13 need as much protein as a man. Boys from 14–19 need more.

24. Girls of 11 need as much as women of 30. Children need proteins in summer, although they are said to be "heating." Cool the children by proper radiation, not by protein starvation. (See "Air," par. 3.)

25. To be sure of vitamins, use some fresh raw food (fruit, etc.) every day.

No. 3. AIR

1. The important points about ordinary air relate to its oxygen, nitrogen, carbonic acid, water vapor, temperature, circulation. We use air for (a) cooling, (b) breathing. Normal air consists of about one-fifth oxygen, four-fifths nitrogen and four parts in 10,000 carbonic acid. The water vapor varies very much.

2. We are like internal combustion engines (see "Food,"

APPENDIX

par. 16) in that we need cooling; like an automobile engine, we are cooled by air and water.

3. The skin is our great radiator; the air itself cools our skins directly; and also by evaporating the water (sweat) that we constantly pour out on our skins.

4. We are like engines also in that we use air to help burn our fuel (see "Food," par. 16). We draw the oxygen through our lungs to the blood, which carries the oxygen to all parts of the body, and brings back the carbonic acid.

5. The "smoke" we make is invisible; it is the carbonic acid we throw out from our lungs.

6. The old idea of "good ventilation" largely neglected water vapor, temperature and circulation, and concerned itself chiefly with oxygen, nitrogen and carbonic acid: it recognized breathing but overlooked cooling.

7. The new discoveries (Flügge, Leonard Hill, etc., during the last 8 or 10 years) show that air seldom can be too bad to breathe: it is very often too bad for successful cooling.

8. This means that ordinary "bad air" is not bad on account of its effects on the lungs, but on account of its effects on the skin.

9. Thus, experimentally, men in "foul" air, suffering headache, drowsiness, etc. (the result of bad ventilation in an airtight room), were allowed to breathe good air through tubes leading to the outside of the room. They were not helped by it. Men, outside the room, in good air, were forced to breathe the foul air through tubes. They were not hurt by it.

10. True it is theoretically possible, in a really airtight room, to use up the oxygen in breathing and fill the room with carbonic acid thrown out from the lungs.

11. But our houses and rooms are not airtight: oxygen

will pass in through the walls themselves, if no windows or doors are open: carbonic acid will pass out through the walls. This is especially true in winter, when the temperatures inside and out differ much.

12. Therefore "bad air," which gives headaches, makes people drowsy, etc., is *not* bad from lack of oxygen, or from too much carbonic acid.

13. "Bad air" is bad from too much humidity, too great heat, or both. The victims of the Black Hole of Calcutta died of "heat stroke," not from lack of oxygen or too much carbonic acid. Suppose you run an automobile without any cooling device! Exactly similar is the effect of too much heat or too much humidity, or both, on the human engine.

14. In winter, most houses are too dry. This means excessive evaporation from the body, chilling it, and the house must be heated excessively (to 70 or 75 degrees Fahrenheit) to make up. Evaporating water in the house in winter to raise the humidity from 30 per cent. (now usual) to 60 per cent. (the proper figure) reduces the temperature necessary for comfort to 60 degrees Fahrenheit; and saves coal.

15. In summer, humidity, as well as heat, is too high as a rule. These are hard to control, but the "heat and humidity blanket" which we ourselves make by warming up the air immediately around our own bodies with our own heat and saturating it with our own evaporated sweat can be dissipated by a breeze, an electric fan, or moving about gently. In winter outdoors, we keep our "heat and humidity blanket" close to our skins by our clothing.

16. Children, especially babies, suffer from heat and humidity and for health in summer require light clothing or none, and circulation of air. In winter they need warm, loose clothing.

APPENDIX

No. 4. MEDICAL SUPERVISION OF SCHOOLS

1. Medical supervision of schools means a physician watching over the children, to find where they are weak in their bodies; and to prevent outbreaks of infectious diseases; just as the teacher watches over them to find where the children are weak in their studies; and to prevent disorder.

2. It is true that every teacher should watch the children for evident bodily defects, poor sight, deafness, sickness; and should report these to the principal, or school board for action. But teachers are not trained medical men and cannot be expected to do such work perfectly.

3. The best system of medical school supervision consists in having a full-time physician, expert in this work, with two trained nurse assistants.* Such supervision has two main purposes: I. to (a) discover, and (b) prevent the spread of, infectious diseases; II. to (a) discover, and (b) provide for the correction of, physical defects. But it also helps in —

(a) the discovery of mental peculiarities of the children,
(b) the discovery of unsanitary conditions in the school,
(c) the provision of the best seating, lighting, heating, and other similar matters,
(d) the promotion of cleanliness, order and decency.

This method 1. prevents epidemics,
2. promotes general health,
3. makes a safe, sanitary school.

4. Where a full-time physician specialist cannot be secured, part time of private practising physicians helps; but full-time nurses should be employed as well.

5. Where only one inspection can be secured during a school year, it should be conducted at the opening of the fall term; if two, at the opening of the fall term, and after the Christmas holidays. These single inspections —

* This is the proportion for a population of 20,000.

(a) prevent carrying over vacation epidemics into the schools,

(b) help to detect the more obvious defects and disabilities of the children.

They do not aid in the discovery of epidemics during the school term; nor in the detection of the defects or disabilities developing after attendance at school has begun.

6. The employment of school nurses alone, without any physician as supervisor, accomplishes a good deal in the direction of cleanliness, the following up of obvious cases of disease, defect, or disability, and helps in truancy. But it neither prevents epidemics nor promotes health, mental efficiency, or general sanitation in a thorough-going way.

7. Emergency medical supervision is conducted in epidemics, to detect infected children and protect the others. This is the best method for getting rid of the disease and it does this without closing the schools: it can be done in any school, at any time, without cost, on application to the State Board of Health.

8. Medical school supervision should be supplemented by pre-school supervision; that is, supervision of prospective scholars, children now under school age who will later go to school; and by instruction to mothers before and after the birth of their children, so that the children will not have so many defects and disabilities to correct later.

No. 1. Germs and Disease, should be taught in ALL grades.

No. 2. Food and Water, may be taught in whole or in part to all grades.

No. 3. Air, should be taught in the sixth and higher grades.

No. 4. Medical School Supervision, should be taught in the eighth and higher grades.

PUBLIC HEALTH IN AMERICA

An Arno Press Collection

Ackerknecht, Erwin H[einz]. **Malaria In the Upper Mississippi Valley: 1760-1900.** 1945

Bowditch, Henry I[ngersoll]. **Consumption In New England Or, Locality One of Its Chief Causes and Is Consumption Contagious, Or Communicated By One Person to Another In Any Manner?** 1862/1864. Two Vols. in One.

Buck, Albert H[enry] (Editor). **A Treatise On Hygiene and Public Health.** 1879. Two Vols.

Boston Medical Commission. **The Sanitary Condition of Boston: The Report of a Medical Commission.** 1875

Budd, William. **Typhoid Fever:** Its Nature, Mode of Spreading, and Prevention. 1931

Chapin, Charles V[alue]. **A Report On State Public Health Work,** Based On a Survey of State Boards of Health: Made Under the Direction of the Council on Health and Public Instruction of the American Medical Association. [1915]

Davis, Michael M[arks], Jr. and Andrew R[obert] Warner. **Dispensaries:** Their Management and Development. 1918

Dublin, Louis I[srael] and Alfred J. Lotka. **The Money Value of a Man.** 1930

Dunglison, Robley. **Human Health.** 1844

Emerson, Haven. **Local Health Units for the Nation.** 1945

Emerson, Haven. **A Monograph On the Epidemic of Poliomyelitis (Infantile Paralysis) In New York City In 1916.** 1917

Fish, Hamilton. **Report of the Select Committee of the Senate of the United States On the Sickness and Mortality On Board Emigrant Ships.** 1854

Frost, Wade Hampton. **The Papers of Wade Hampton Frost, M.D.:** A Contribution to Epidemiological Method. 1941

Gardner, Mary Sewall. **Public Health Nursing.** 1916

Greenwood, Major. **Epidemics and Crowd Diseases:** An Introduction to the Study of Epidemiology. 1935

Greenwood, Major. **Medical Statistics From Graunt to Farr.** 1948

Hartley, Robert M. **An Historical, Scientific and Practical Essay On Milk, As an Article of Human Sustenance:** With a Consideration of the Effects Consequent Upon the Unnatural Methods of Producing It for the Supply of Large Cities. 1842

Hill, Hibbert Winslow. **The New Public Health.** 1916

Knopf, S. Adolphus. **Tuberculosis As a Disease of the Masses & How To Combat It.** 1908

MacNutt, J[oseph] Scott. **A Manual for Health Officers.** 1915

Richards, Ellen H. [Swallow]. **Euthenics:** The Science of Controllable Environment. 1910

Richardson, Joseph G[ibbons]. **Long Life and How To Reach It.** 1886

Rumsey, Henry Wyldbore. **Essays On State Medicine.** 1856

Shryock, Richard Harrison. **National Tuberculosis Association 1904-1954:** A Study of the Voluntary Health Movement In the United States. 1957

Simon, John. **Filth-Diseases and Their Prevention.** 1876

Sternberg, George M[iller]. **Sanitary Lessons of the War and Other Papers.** 1912

Straus, Lina Gutherz. **Disease In Milk:** The Remedy Pasteurization. The Life Work of Nathan Straus. 1917

Wanklyn, J[ames] Alfred and Ernest Theophron Chapman. **Water Analysis:** A Practical Treatise on the Examination of Potable Water. 1884

Whipple, George C. **State Sanitation:** A Review of the Work of the Massachusetts State Board of Health. 1917. Two Vols. in One.

Selections From Public Health Reports and Papers Presented at the Meetings of the American Public Health Association (1873-1883). 1977

Selections From Public Health Reports and Papers Presented at the Meetings of the American Public Health Association (1884-1907). 1977

Animalcular and Cryptogamic Theories On the Origins of Fevers. 1977

The Carrier State. 1977

Clean Water and the Health of the Cities. 1977

The First American Medical Association Reports On Public Hygiene In American Cities. 1977

Selections from the Health-Education Series. 1977

Health In the Southern United States. 1977

Health In the Twentieth Century. 1977

The Health of Women and Children. 1977

Minutes and Proceedings from the First, Second, Third and Fourth National Quarantine and Sanitary Conventions. 1977. Four Vols. in Two.

Selections from the Journal of the Massachusetts Association of Boards of Health (1891-1904). 1977

Sewering the Cities. 1977

Smallpox In Colonial America. 1977

Yellow Fever Studies. 1977

NORTHERN ILLINOIS UNIVERSITY

3 1211 01561492 4